Pᴀɪɴ Mᴇᴅɪᴄɪɴᴇ
Pocketpedia

PAIN MEDICINE
POCKETPEDIA

Hyung S. Kim, MD
Pain Physiatrist,
VA Greater Los Angeles Healthcare System,
Los Angeles, California

David E. Fish, MD, MPH
Associate Professor of Orthopaedic Surgery and
Associate Program Director,
Pain Medicine (PM&R) Fellowship Program
David Geffen School of Medicine at UCLA,
Los Angeles, California

Howard Choi, MD, MPH
Attending Physician
North Shore-Long Island Jewish Health System
New Hyde Park, New York

Wolters Kluwer | Lippincott Williams & Wilkins
Health

Philadelphia · Baltimore · New York · London
Buenos Aires · Hong Kong · Sydney · Tokyo

Acquisitions Editor: Robert Hurley
Product Manager: Dave Murphy
Marketing Manager: Lisa Lawrence
Manufacturing Manager: Benjamin Rivera
Design Manager: Doug Smock
Printer: RR Donnelley, Shenzhen, China

International Standard Book Number ISBN 0-7817-7218-4, 9-780-7817-7218-1

Printed in China

Library of Congress Cataloging-in-Publication Data

Kim, Hyung S., author.
  Pain medicine pocketpedia / Hyung S. Kim, MD, Pain Physiatrist, VA
Greater Los Angeles Healthcare System, Los Angeles, California, David E.
Fish, MD, MPH, Associate Professor of Orthopaedic Surgery and Associate
Program Director, Pain Medicine (PM&R) Fellowship Program, David Geffen
School of Medicine at UCLA, Los Angeles, California, Howard Choi, MD,
MPH, Attending Physician, North Shore-Long Island Jewish Health System,
New Hyde Park, New York.
     p. ; cm.
  Includes bibliographical references and index.
  ISBN-13: 978-0-7817-7218-1 (alk. paper)
  ISBN-10: 0-7817-7218-4 (alk. paper)
  1. Pain–Treatment–Handbooks, manuals, etc.   2. Analgesia–Handbooks,
manuals, etc. I. Fish, David E., author. II. Choi, Howard, author. III.
Title.
  [DNLM: 1. Pain–therapy–Handbooks.   2. Analgesics–therapeutic
use–Handbooks.   3. Pain–diagnosis–Handbooks. WL 39]
  RB127.K428 2011
  616′.0472–dc22

                                                       2010053245

DISCLAIMER
    Care has been taken to confirm the accuracy of the information present and to describe generally accepted practices. However, the authors, editors, and publisher are not responsible for errors or omissions or for any consequences from application of the information in this book and make no warranty, expressed or implied, with respect to the currency, completeness, or accuracy of the contents of the publication. Application of this information in a particular situation remains the professional responsibility of the practitioner; the clinical treatments described and recommended may not be considered absolute and universal recommendations.
    The authors, editors, and publisher have exerted every effort to ensure that drug selection and dosage set forth in this text are in accordance with the current recommendations and practice at the time of publication. However, in view of ongoing research, changes in government regulations, and the constant flow of information relating to drug therapy and drug reactions, the reader is urged to check the package insert for each drug for any change in indications and dosage and for added warnings and precautions. This is particularly important when the recommended agent is a new or infrequently employed drug.
    Some drugs and medical devices presented in this publication have Food and Drug Administration (FDA) clearance for limited use in restricted research settings. It is the responsibility of the health care provider to ascertain the FDA status of each drug or device planned for use in their clinical practice.

To purchase additional copies of this book, call our customer service department at **(800) 638-3030** or fax orders to **(301) 223-2320**. International customers should call **(301) 223-2300**.

Visit Lippincott Williams & Wilkins on the Internet: http://www.lww.com. Lippincott Williams & Wilkins customer service representatives are available from 8:30 am to 6:00 pm, EST.

CONTENTS

FOREWORD

Despite its ubiquitous nature, pain is not well covered in the current medical curriculum. Part of the problem may be that pain has yet to receive a clear definition, even if organizations such as the International Association for the Study of Pain have attempted to describe pain as an "unpleasant sensory and emotional experience associated with actual or potential tissue damage." With the recent emergence of pain medicine as a distinct field of its own and demand by the public that pain be better addressed, the importance of pain medicine will only grow.

Pain Medicine Pocketpedia was written as a quick, portable reference book for select topics in this emerging, exciting field. Understanding of the nature of pain and treatments for various pain states are rapidly evolving. It is hoped that this small book be able to assist busy students and practitioners understand and manage those suffering from pain as it is understood today.

Rene Calliet, MD
Professor Emeritus,
Keck School of Medicine of the
University of Southern California
and Clinical Professor Emeritus,
Physical Medicine & Rehabilitation,
David Geffen School of Medicine at UCLA

CONTRIBUTORS

Dixie R. Aragaki, MD Associate Director, PM&R Residency Program, VA Greater Los Angeles Healthcare System (GLAHS) and Assistant Professor of Medicine, David Geffen School of Medicine at UCLA, Los Angeles, California

Arash Asher, MD Director, Cancer Survivorship & Rehabilitation, Samuel Oschin Comprehensive Cancer Institute at Cedars-Sinai Medical Center, Los Angeles, California

Ariel Baria, NP Coordinator, Inpatient Chronic Pain Service, VA Greater Los Angeles Healthcare System, Los Angeles, California,

Ervin Bernotus, MD Private Practice in PM&R, Pain Medicine and Spinal Cord Injury Medicine, Sarasota, Florida

J. Bren Boston, MD Interventional Physiatrist, Los Angeles, California

Eric Y. Chang, MD Clinical fellow, Pain Medicine, Department of Anesthesiology and Perioperative Care, UC Irvine School of Medicine, Irvine, California

Beny Charchian, MD, MS Clinical fellow, Pain Medicine (PM&R), UCLA/VA Greater Los Angeles Healthcare System, Los Angeles, California

C. Joey Chang, MD Staff Physician, Dusk to Dawn Urgent Care Centers, Paramount, California

Alan Chen, MD Interventional Physiatrist, Cascade Orthopaedics, Auburn, Washington

Heather Rachel Davids, MD Division Head, Pain Medicine, Mercy Medical Group, Sacramento, California

Jeffrey T. Ho, DO MS Assistant Professor, Physical Medicine and Rehabilitation, University of California, Irvine; Rehab Associates Medical Group, Long Beach Memorial Medical Center, Long Beach, California

Marilyn S. Jacobs, PhD Clinical Faculty in Psychology, David Geffen School of Medicine at UCLA, Los Angeles, California

Antoine Jones, MD Interventional Physiatrist, Seattle, Washington

Woojae Kim, MD Resident, PM&R, UCLA/VA Greater Los Angeles Healthcare System, Los Angeles, California

Ira Kornbluth, MD Interventional Physiatrist, Baltimore, Maryland

Daniel B. Marcus, MD Medical Director, Rehabilitation Services, Palo Alto Medical Foundation Santa Cruz, California

Anh Quan Nguyen, DO Chief, Chronic Pain Service, Kaiser Permanente Orange Medical Center, Orange, California

Sanjog S. Pangarkar, MD Director, Inpatient Pain Service, VA GLAHS and Assistant Professor of Medicine, David Geffen School of Medicine at UCLA, Los Angeles, California

Quynh G. Pham, MD Director, Pain Medicine (PM&R) Fellowship Program and PM&R Residency Program, VA GLAHS and Associate Professor of Medicine, David Geffen School of Medicine at UCLA, Los Angeles, California

Walter Van Vort, MD Attending Psychiatrist, VA Greater Los Angeles Healthcare System

Milena D. Zirovich, MD Attending physician, PM&R Pain Medicine, VA Greater Los Angeles Health Care System, Los Angeles, California

Part One
Fundamentals and Evaluation

Ch.1: A VERY BRIEF HISTORY OF PAIN MEDICINE

Pain has plagued humanity since antiquity. The search for relief from pain is no less old. Primitive therapies for pain included rubbing afflicted body parts, exposing painful areas to cold water or heat from the sun or fire, and mystical rituals. Some ancient cultures developed rich pharmacopiae, including medicines derived from the willow plant (salicylates) and the opium poppy.

Rene Descartes (1596–1650) is credited with the idea that pain is transmitted from the periphery to the brain via "nerve filaments." In the early 19th century, morphine was identified as a key active ingredient in opium. Its use was greatly enhanced a few decades later with the development of the hypodermic needle and syringe. In 1894, Max von Frey described specific receptors involved in the transmission of pain signals. In 1920, Head and Rivers proposed that the thalamus was the "pain center" and that the cerebral cortex could inhibit pain. Advances in the treatment of pain during the early 20th century included the development of acetaminophen, phenylbutazone, and the semisynthetic opioid analgesics derived from morphine (such as heroin, hydromorphone, and meperidine), as well as the development of the first spinal injections for pain.

During the mid 20th century, John Bonica described the psychological and drug abuse problems of the chronic pain patient and advocated for a multidisciplinary approach to treating chronic pain. In 1965, Melzack and Wall published their landmark paper on gate-control theory, which proposed a rational scientific mechanism to explain how the perception of pain may be modulated. Over the last few decades, advances in treatment have included new psychological approaches, transcutaneous electrical nerve stimulation, fluoroscopically guided interventions, implantable devices such as the spinal cord stimulator and intrathecal pump, and a panoply of new drugs.

Pain medicine grew rapidly as a field during the latter half of the 20th century. Pain Medicine is now formally recognized by the American Board of Medical Specialties as a medical subspecialty in its own right. Continued growth and maturation of the field is anticipated for the forseeable future.

Ref: Loeser JD, et al., eds. *Bonica's Management of Pain*, 3rd ed. Philadelphia, LWW, 2001; **Melzack R, Wall P**. Pain mechanisms: A new theory. *Science* 1965;150:971; **Raj PP**. *Pain medicine: A comprehensive review*. Mosby-Year Book, 1996.

Ch.2: DEFINITIONS AND EPIDEMIOLOGY

Pain is "an unpleasant sensory and emotional experience associated with actual or potential tissue damage or described in terms of such damage. Pain is always subjective." (International Association for the Study of Pain).

Whereas *acute pain* is not *primarily* due to psychopathology or environmental influences, in chronic pain these influences play a prominent role. John Bonica, a pioneer in pain medicine, believed that chronic pain is pain persisting "a month beyond the usual course of a disease or a reasonable time for an injury to heal or associated with a chronic pathological process . . ." The term "chronic pain syndrome" was introduced in the 1970s to describe cases of intractable pain complaints out of proportion to the objective findings, with significant psychological overlay.

    Paresthesia is an abnormal sensation, whether evoked or spontaneous, while dysesthesia is an unpleasant parasthesia. *Hyperalgesia* is a subset of dysesthesia where there is an increased response to a stimulus which is normally painful, whereas *allodynia* is pain evoked by a stimulus that is normally not painful. *Static allodynia* is allodynia from a static stimulus (e.g., light pressure), while *dynamic allodynia* is an allodynia resulting from a dynamic stimulus (e.g., stroking with cotton wool). *Hyperesthesia* is an increased sensitivity to stimulation (with or without pain). *Thermal hyperesthesia* describes hyperesthesia to normally non-nociceptive warm or cold stimuli. *Hypoesthesia* is a decreased sensitivity to stimulation. *Hyperpathia* is an increase in painful response to a stimulus, especially a repetitive stimulus.

Epidemiology - Pain is universal to the human experience. In the United States, it appears that 20 to 30% of the general population experience chronic or recurring pain (Weiner, 2007). Approximately 2/3 of these people have had pain for more than 5 years (Loeser, 2001). The cost of chronic pain has been estimated to be as high as $100 billion a year in the United States.

Ref: Weiner K. Pain issues: Pain is an epidemic. American Academy of Pain Management. Available from: http://www.aapainmanage.org accessed January 26, 2007; **Loeser JD et al, eds.** *Bonica's management of pain.* Philadelphia: LWW, 2001.

Ch.3: ANATOMY AND PHYSIOLOGY OF PAIN

Basic pathways of nociceptive pain - Peripheral pain stimuli are detected by primary afferent *nociceptors*, which transmit pain centrally via unmyelinated C fibers or thinly myelinated Aδ fibers.

Pain fiber	Diameter	myelination	Conduction velocity
C	< 2 μm	unmyelinated	2 m/s
Aδ	2–5 μm	thinly myelinated	6–30 m/s

The cell bodies of the primary afferent nociceptors are located in the dorsal root ganglia (DRG) and their fibers terminate on second order neurons in the dorsal horn of the spinal cord.

Lissauer's tract consists of smaller fibers that congregate together prior to synapsing in the dorsal-most layers of the dorsal horn. Most nociceptive input from the periphery transmits to Rexed layers I (marginal layer), II (substantia gelatinosa) or V (the deepest portion of the nucleus proprius, which consists of Rexed layers III-V). Excitatory neuromediators related to pain transmission identified in the dorsal horn have included glutamate, substance P, calcitonin gene-related peptide (CGRP), and bradykinin. The aforementioned dorsal horn layers, in turn, project to the ascending pathways. Spinal cord pathways that have been implicated in ascending nociceptive pain signal transmission include the spinothalamic tract, spinoreticular tract, spinomesencephalic tract and postsynaptic dorsal column tract.

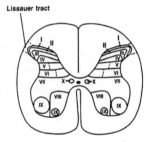

Figure 3a Rexed laminae.

The spinothalamic tract is the most important of the ascending tracts in relation to pain transmission. Most of its neurons arise from Rexed lamina I. Along with fibers arising from laminae II and V, this pathway (termed the neospinothalamic pathway) transmits the sensory and discriminative aspects of pain to the lateral thalamus and sensorimotor cortex. Neurons residing in deeper Rexed laminae (VI, IX) contribute to spinothalamic tract fibers projecting to the medial thalamus, reticular formation, periaqueductal gray, hypothalamus, and other areas of the limbic system. This pathway (the paleospinothalamic tract) is associated with the affective aspects of pain.

Other portions of the brain involved with higher nociceptive signal processing (cingulate cortex, lentiform nucleus, insula, anterior cingulate, and prefrontal cortex) have been demonstrated on functional MRI and PET studies (Gybels, 1985).

Visceral pain is transmitted from nociceptors in the visceral organs to the spinal cord via visceral afferents. The cell bodies are located in the dorsal root ganglia and the fibers travel together with sympathetic and parasympathetic axons. Visceral nociceptive C fibers converge in many Rexed laminae including I, II, IV, V, and X. The second order neurons then transmit the signals to the brain via the spinothalamic tracts. Viscero-somatic convergence refers to the convergence of visceral and somatic afferents at the spinal cord dorsal horn

6

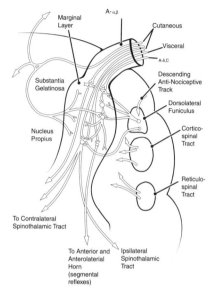

Figure 3b Dorsal horn.

before relaying signals are transmitted to the brain. The higher central nervous system (CNS), however, interprets signals as coming from a dermatomal level, without discriminating between somatic or visceral origin.

The sympathetic nervous system likely plays an important role in nociception, although its exact contribution is not yet completely understood. It is known that the sympathetic system plays a critical role in global behavioral response to noxious input, i.e., the fight or flight response.

Descending pathways that modulate pain have been postulated to exist since the 1960s. Endogenous opioid-mediated pathways involving the periaqueductal gray and other CNS areas have been experimentally demonstrated. In addition, there are descending noradrenergic tracts in the dorsolateral funiculus that can be stimulated to produce analgesia (e.g., by clonidine, an α2 agonist). Noradrenergic neurons associated with the locus ceruleus also mediate behavioral responses to noxious input and are hypothesized to modulate the pain response indirectly as well. Serotonergic systems projecting from the nucleus raphe magnus via the dorsolateral funiculus to the spinal cord are also involved in descending pain modulation.

Peripheral sensitization refers to a process whereby the peptides released secondary to pain and inflammation result in sensitization of high-threshold nociceptors. Nociceptor activation initiates a process that modifies responses to further sensory stimuli. For example, a relatively benign noxious stimulus such as a skin scratch initiates a peripheral inflammation cascade that reduces the threshold for response of the nociceptor to subsequent sensory stimuli.

Nociceptive stimulation results in inflammatory responses with release of peptides such as substance P, CGRP, and neurokinin A from the peripheral terminals of nociceptive afferent fibers. These peptides in turn modify the excitability of sensory and sympathetic nerve fibers, induce vasodilation and extravasation of plasma proteins, and promote the release of further chemical mediators. These interactions result in a mixture of inflammatory mediators, including serotonin, bradykinin, substance P, histamine, cytokines, nitric oxide, and products from the cyclooxygenase and lipoxygenase pathways of arachidonic acid metabolism (Woolf, 1993).

Central sensitization refers to neural plasticity displayed by the central neural structures involved with nociception, with resultant recruitment of previously subthreshold synaptic inputs to nociceptive neurons, generating an increased or augmented action potential output (Latremoliere, 2009). Glutamate is the primary excitatory neurotransmitter of the CNS and is normally released by pain-signaling afferent neurons as they synapse on central pain pathways in the spinal cord. The resultant persistent release of glutamate leads to activation of N-methyl-D-aspartate (NMDA) receptors. NMDA receptor activation plays a crucial role in mediating the phenomenon of "wind-up" pain, a state in which spinal neurons become hyperresponsive to repetitive painful stimulation. Allodynia and hyperalgesia, two hallmarks of neuropathic pain, are expressions of "wind-up" pain. Agents with NMDA antagonist activity such as methadone and ketamine have shown some success in controlling chronic nonmalignant pain (Dickenson, 1990; Kiefer, 2007).

Examples where central sensitization is thought to be involved include neuropathic and inflammatory pain, migraine headache, irritable bowel syndrome, and fibromyalgia. In some cases, both peripheral and central sensitization may play a role, as seen in complex regional pain syndrome.

There are two forms of second-order spinal neurons that are involved in central sensitization: (1) nociceptive-specific neurons which respond only to nociceptive stimuli and (2) wide-dynamic range (WDR) neurons which respond to both nociceptive and non-nociceptive afferent stimuli. In general, WDR neurons are more highly sensitized than nociceptive-specific neurons because both nociceptive and non-nociceptive peripheral nerves often converge on the same WDR neuron. Hence, once sensitized by ongoing nociceptive impulses from peripheral nerves, WDR neurons will respond to non-nociceptive stimuli as intensely as to nociceptive stimuli. This is how, for instance, light touch might be experienced as pain (allodynia).

Gate-control theory of pain - Melzack and Wall published their gate-control theory in Science in 1965. They postulated that peripheral afferent large fibers (transmitting non-painful signals) and small fibers (transmitting painful signals) project to a "gate control" system in the dorsal horn of the spinal cord, consisting of the substantia gelatinosa and transmission (T) cells. Large fiber activity reduces T cell activity ("closes the gate"), while small fibers increase T cell activity ("open the gate"). When T cell activity exceeds a threshold, the "action system" is activated, resulting in the experience of pain and complex behavioral responses. Higher CNS pathways (neocortical and brainstem) evaluate the sensory input based on past experiences, influence the gate, and modulate the response.

The gate-control theory has served as the most widely accepted model of pain, underscoring the interaction between the physical and psychological components of pain, and providing insight into the treatment of pain (e.g., explains the relief achieved by rubbing painful areas). The theory precipitated the development of spinal cord stimulators (which were intended to stimulate A-β fibers to "close" the dorsal horn gate), although recent research suggests that other mechanisms are operating sequentially or simultaneously. Indeed, more recent models point to pathological pain pathways and central neuromatrices which are much more complex than the model presented by the gate-control theory.

Ref: Gybels JM. Neurosurgical treatment of persistent pain: Physiological and pathological mechanisms of human pain. In Gildenberg PL, ed: Pain and headache, vol. 11. Basel, Karger, 1985; **Woolf CJ, Chong MS**. Preemptive analgesia: treating postoperative pain by preventing the establishment of central sensitization. *Anes Anal* 1993;77:362; **Latremoliere A, Woolf CJ**. Central Sensitization: A Generator of Pain Hypersensitivity by Central Neural Plasticity. *J Pain* 2009;10:895; **Dickenson AH**. A cure for wind up: NMDA receptor antagonists as potential analgesics. *Trends Pharmacol Sci* 1990;11:307; **Kiefer RT et al.** Complete recovery from intractable complex regional pain syndrome, CRPS-type I, following anesthetic ketamine and midazolam. *Pain Pract* 2007;7:147; **Melzack R, Wall PD**. Pain mechanisms: A new theory, *Science* 1965;150:971.

Figure credits: 3a. Courtesy of **Ballantyne JC**. *The MGH Handbook of Pain Management*, 3rd ed. Philadelphia, LWW, 2006, with permission; **3b.** Courtesy of **Loeser JD, et al.,** eds. *Bonica's Management of Pain*, 3rd ed. Philadelphia, LWW, 2001, with permission.

Ch.4: EVALUATION AND MEASUREMENT OF PAIN

Proper pain management requires an adequate evaluation, and an etiological diagnosis of the pain should always be explored. The evaluation should include a specific history of the pain, including location, radiation, intensity, aggravating and alleviating factors, and temporal descriptors (e.g., frequency, chronicity). Patterns of referred pain (below) should always be considered:

pain source	region of pain referral
upper cervical facets	occiput, vertex, frontal head
lower cervical facets	shoulder, neck pain
aortic dissection	mid back
pancreas	mid back
liver capsule	shoulder pain
kidney	low thoracic/lumbar pain
prostate/uterus	low back pain
lumbar facets	buttock, groin, thigh, calf pain
sacroiliac joints	buttock, groin, thigh, calf pain

Evaluation generally includes detailed physical examinations including provocative tests, lab and imaging tests, and referrals to psychologists when appropriate. Frequently, the patient has already seen many physicians prior to seeing a pain specialist, and will carry many diagnoses already. A careful review of these diagnoses is critical.

Although pain is subjective and problematic to quantify, the measurement of pain using various scales can nonetheless aid in the assessment of treatment effectiveness. Examples of pain measures include the visual analog scale, numerical ratings scale, verbal rating scales, picture scales (e.g., Wong-Baker Faces Pain Rating Scale) and the McGill Pain Questionnaire.

The *visual analog scale* (VAS, see figure below) of pain intensity is typically 10 cm in length and has word descriptions on either end, such as "no pain" and "worst pain."

no pain ├────────────────────────────────┤ worst pain

The VAS is sensitive to treatment interventions and has good reliability within a single patient (although comparisons between patients are more difficult to interpret). A score of ≤30 mm is considered "mild," 31–69 mm "moderate," and ≥70 mm "severe" pain. The minimal clinically significant distance to correspond to treatment improvement has been reported to be 13 mm (10–17 mm 95% C.I.) in acute traumatic pain (Todd, 1996), and does not vary significantly with age, gender, etiology of pain, or severity of pain (Kelly, 2001).

The *numerical rating scale* is an ordinal 0–10 scale, vs. the VAS, which is continuous. Many variations, including verbal rating scales, exist. The NIH Pain Consortium uses a 0–10 scale where 1–3 represents mild pain (annoying, but interfering little with activities of daily living [ADLs]), 4–6 is moderate pain (interfering significantly with ADLs), and 7–10 is severe pain (disabling, unable to perform ADLs; McCaffery, 1993). Numeric scales are superior in retrospective reliability to the VAS for recalled chronic pain. Scales using facial drawings (e.g., the Wong-Baker Faces Pain Rating Scale used by the NIH Pain Consortium) can be useful when there are age (children), cognitive, or language issues.

Overall, unidimensional scales are valid and easy to administer, but risk oversimplifying the pain complaint and do not adequately address the affective component of pain.

The *McGill Pain Questionnaire* is a multidimensional pain measurement tool developed by Melzack and colleagues at McGill University in the 1970s. There are 4 sections: 1) location of pain: the patient marks areas afflicted by pain on a diagram of the body using "I" (internal pain), "E" (external) or "EI" (external and internal); 2) scores for the sensory, affective, and evaluative dimensions of pain, determined by the pain rating index: the patient selects from a series of 78 descriptors (e.g., pounding, fearful, pulling, sharp) in 20 groups in the index; only one word per group at maximum is circled; 3) pattern of pain (e.g., continuous, intermittent, transient, and alleviating/aggravating factors); and 4) present pain intensity, measured on a 0–5 scale.

There are shortened and extended versions of the McGill Pain Questionnaire and versions in other languages. Lack of sophistication with language sometimes limits the utility of this questionnaire. The Short-form McGill Pain Questionnaire (1987) is comprised of a VAS, the present pain intensity from the long-form, and 15 pain descriptor words (11 sensory and four affective words) scored from 0–3 in intensity.

Ref: Todd KH. Clinical vs. statistical significance in the assessment of pain relief. *Ann Emerg Med J* 1996;27:439; **Kelly AM.** The minimum clinically significant difference in VAS pain score does not differ with severity of pain. *Emerg Med J* 2001;18:205; **McCaffery M, et al.** Pain: Clinical manual for nursing practice. Baltimore, Mosby, 1993; **Melzack R.** The McGill Pain Questionnaire: major properties and scoring methods. *Pain* 1975;1:277.

Ch.5: HISTORY AND EXAM FOR SPINE-RELATED PAIN

A proper history helps to determine the differential diagnosis. Key potential pain generators include the discal fibrous ring and the spinal nerve roots. When the fibrous ring is stretched, there is axial pain. When the anulus breaks and the nucleus pulposus extrudes (chemically or physically affecting the nerve roots), a radicular pain can ensue. Notably, pain radiating below the knee is more likely to represent a true radiculopathy than pain radiating to the posterior thigh.

Red flags on history suggestive of an underlying systemic disease responsible for the spinal pain include advanced age, history of cancer, history of IV drug use, fever, unexplained weight loss, and failure of bed rest to relieve the pain.

Differential diagnosis of acute spinal pain

Fracture - Spinous process
Pars interarticularis (spondylolysis)
Vertebral body (osteoporotic, neoplastic [primary: multiple myeloma, osteosarcoma; metastatic: lung, breast, prostate, kidney, thyroid], traumatic [typically thoracolumbar])

Infection - Osteomyelitis (tuberculosis/Pott's disease)
Discitis
Epidural abscess (staphylococcus, streptococcus, pseudomonas)
Herpes zoster (shingles)

Soft tissue - Muscle strain
Neural elements (radiculitis, spinal cord, arachnoiditis, meningeal irritation)
Disc herniation, sequestration
Ligamentous disruption/injury

Other/medical - Genitourinary (kidney stone, pyelonephritis)
Gastrointestinal (gallstone, pancreatitis)
Vascular (abdominal aortic aneurysm, aortic dissection)
Retroperitoneal process/bleed
Bone infarct (sickle cell disease)

Differential diagnosis of subacute/chronic spinal pain

Somatic nociceptive - Degenerative disc disease
Ligamentous (anterior longitudinal ligament, posterior longitudinal ligament, interspinous ligament)
Facet arthropathy
Spondylolisthesis (L4–5 common in degenerative, L5-S1 most common in young acquired/congenital)
Rheumatological disorder (Ankylosing spondylitis, rheumatoid arthritis)
Sacroiliac joint dysfunction
Piriformis syndrome
Myofascial pain
Post-surgical changes (failed back surgery, scar tissue)

Visceral referred pain - Gastrointestinal (bowel distention, chronic pancreatitis)
Genitourinary
Cardiovascular

Neuropathic - Radiculopathy, spinal stenosis, arachnoiditis, neoplasm

Psychogenic - Somatization, depression, anxiety, malingering

Physical exam

Observation of gait and posture - A forward stooped gait may suggest hip flexion contractures or compensatory positioning to alleviate symptoms of lumbar spinal stenosis.

Inspection - The normal spine has four postural curves: cervical lordosis, thoracic kyphosis, lumbar lordosis, and sacral kyphosis. Reduced curvature may be secondary to cervical or lumbar paraspinal muscle spasm. A loss of lumbar lordosis may be indicative of disc or vertebral body collapse. Thoracic kyphosis or "dowager's hump" can be due to thoracic compression fractures. Increased lumbar lordosis may be seen with high grade spondylolisthesis or in the very obese.

Additionally, scoliosis should be noted because chronic rotation and lateral curves may lead to spinal stenosis and narrowing of lateral recesses as well as intervertebral foraminal stenosis leading to radiculopathy. If Adam's forward bending test (a screening test used in grade schools) reveals asymmetrical rise of the thorax upon forward flexion, scoliosis should be suspected.

Palpation - Spinous processes, paraspinal muscles, iliolumbar and sacroiliac ligaments, iliac crests, posterior superior iliac spine, greater trochanters, and piriformis muscles should be palpated. Midline tenderness could reflect a disc problem, bone neoplasm, or bone fracture. Pain on percussion can be a sign of a potentially serious problem such as a metastasis or infection. Tenderness over the sacroiliac joint is the leading presenting symptom for sacroiliac joint dysfunction. Trigger points can be identified within muscles by exquisite tenderness, palpable taut band, twitch sign, and referred pain in a predictable pattern reproducible by deep palpation.

Range of motion testing - Reduced soft tissue flexibility and positions that provoke or alleviate symptoms should be noted in ROM testing. Test for the presence of asymmetrical limitations, e.g., at the hip vs. spine, should also be performed. Tight hamstrings or paraspinal muscles limit flexion, whereas tight hip flexors or facet arthropathy limits extension.

Provocative tests:

Cervical radiculopathy/myelopathy pathology: A literature review by Rubinstein (2006) concluded that, when compatible with the history and other physical findings, a positive Spurling's test, traction/neck distraction, and Valsalva maneuver can be suggestive of cervical radiculopathy (high specificity), while a negative upper limb tension test can help rule it out (high sensitivity). No single test, however, had both high sensitivity and specificity. Methodological problems with the primary studies precluded strong recommendations about the validity and utility of the tests. No studies on the axial compression test met the review's minimal criteria for inclusion.

In a 2003 review, Malanga, et al., found high specificity, low sensitivity, and fair to good interrater reliability for the shoulder abduction, Spurling's, and neck distraction tests. Conclusions about the sensitivity, specificity, or interrater reliability of L'hermitte's sign could not be drawn from the existing literature.

In the ***axial compression test***, the examiner places a caudally directed force on top of the patient's head. Local neck pain suggests cervical spinal degenerative disease, while radiating pain suggests cervical nerve root impingement. Test sensitivity, however, is low (Viikari-Juntura, 1989).

Lhermitte's sign is a reproduction of pain down the spine and legs when a patient's head is flexed at the neck while the patient sits with hips flexed and knees extended. A positive test has been suggested to indicate dural or meningeal irritation or cervical myelopathy, as in multiple sclerosis.

In *Spurling's test*, an axial compressive force is placed on the head with the neck slightly extended, rotated, and laterally flexed towards the symptomatic side. Ipsilateral radicular radiation of pain suggests cervical neuroforaminal narrowing and nerve root irritation.

In a *positive traction/neck distraction test*, lifting the chin and occiput upwards and away from the shoulders relieves pain due to cervical radiculopathy by widening the cervical foramen.

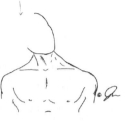

Figure 5a Spurling's test.

For the *Valsalva test*, the patient holds a deep breath while seated and bears down as if to evacuate the bowels. Increased pain during this maneuver indicates increased intrathecal pressure or nerve root irritation. Pain may also occur in the low back, suggesting lumbar nerve root compression.

The *upper limb tension test*, sometimes referred to as the "straight leg test for the arm," is a series of maneuvers designed to place the cervical nerve roots and brachial plexus in various degrees of traction. The patient is placed in the supine position and the following are performed progressively: shoulder girdle depression, glenohumeral abduction, wrist extension, wrist supination, elbow extension, and contralateral neck lateral flexion.

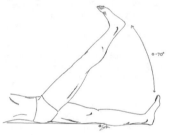

Lumbar facet arthropathy - pain with prolonged standing or hyperextension (e.g., sleeping prone or swimming); pain may go down to the buttock or posterior thigh but not usually below the knee; Stork's test is a common screening test performed via hyperextending a patient standing on one leg while laterally rotating the spine to create pressure at the zygapophysial joint and posterior elements of the affected side creates pain.

Figure 5b Straight leg raise may produce sciatic nerve or lumbosacral nerve root pain. Ankle dorsiflexion may increase tension and referred pain (*Lasegue's sign*).

Discogenic pain - May have positive straight leg raise with a spinal nerve compression; clinical clues of disc herniation-worsening pain with forward flexion/rotation, Valsalva maneuver, prolonged sitting.

Spondylolisthesis - A step-off between sequential spinous processes may be felt during midline

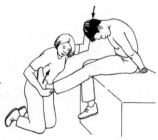

Figure 5c Slump test.

palpation; patients may report pain with excessive forward flexion and/or extension and sometimes have lumbar hyperlordosis with anterior pelvic tilt.

Lumbar spinal stenosis - May be associated with back pain and leg weakness after prolonged standing or walking, relieved by forward flexion (or "pushing on shopping cart" position). Usually no pain with sitting or with seated exercises, e.g., bicycling. Spinal stenosis may be distinguished from vascular claudication if forward flexion of spine when walking up the stairs reduces pain, a phenomena seen in neurogenic but not in vascular claudication.

Lumbosacral radiculopathy - Common tests for suspected lumbosacral radiculopathy include:

Straight leg raise (SLR) test. From the supine position, knee is extended and leg is raised until back or leg pain is elicited. Reproduction of pain at hip angles of 35–70° indicates a positive test. If pain only occurs at >70° of hip flexion, then the hip joint should be suspected as the source of pain. Dorsiflexion of the foot with the leg extended (Lasegue's maneuver) can add additional tension on the root. The crossed SLR is positive if symptoms are reproduced by raising the unaffected (the "good") leg.

Slump test (or sitting root test). The patient sits on the edge of exam table with the legs and hips supported in a neutral position, then leans head and upper body into forward flexion while the knees are extended and ankles are dorsiflexed. Reproducible back pain indicates "long tract" or neural irritation.

The *Kernig/Brudzinski test* is performed with the patient supine and neck flexed. The hip is flexed with knee extended until pain is elicited. If there is relief with flexion of the knee, the test is positive.

Dermatomal or myotomal patterns of symptoms are suggestive of root level involvement; straight leg raise or hyperextension may provoke referred pain via narrowing intervertebral foramen.

Signs and symptoms according to the level:
- L2–4 radiculopathy - lack of patellar reflex or referred pain with femoral nerve stretch (hyperextending hip with knee flexed in prone or lateral decubitus position)
- L5 radiculopathy - weakness of the extensor hallucis longus/dorsiflexors with associated parasthesias in the first dorsal webspace and reduced medial hamstring reflex
- S1 radiculopathy - loss of Achilles reflex, weakness of plantarflexors and hamstrings, gluteal pain and parasthesias in the lateral/plantar foot

The sensitivity and specificity of many physical exam tests in diagnosing lumbosacral radiculopathy are generally low. In one metanalysis, only the straight leg test (SLR) was demonstrated to be sensitive for sciatica due to disc herniation, with a pooled sensitivity of 85% and specificity of 52%, while the crossed SLR was more specific (84%), but less sensitive (30%; Vroomen, 1999). Another review found no tests to have high sensitivity or specificity for radiculopathy (van den Hoogen, 1995).

Sacroiliitis/Sacroiliac joint dysfunction - In the *FABER (or Patrick's) test*, the hip is placed into the Flexion/ABduction/Externally Rotation position while in the supine position. The examiner pushes down with one hand on the flexed knee and the other on the opposite iliac crest to stabilize the pelvis. Pain in the sacroiliac joint region is suggestive of sacroiliac joint pain. Groin or hip pain is suggestive of true hip joint pain.

Gaenslen's test. One leg of the supine patient is flexed at the hip to the chest, while the other hip is allowed to hyperextend off the edge of table. Pain in the hyperextended sacroiliac joint regions marks a positive test and sacroiliac joint pathology.

Gillet's test. Limited iliac crest movement when the ipsilateral hip and knee are flexed at 90 degrees while standing on the opposite limb; iliac crest should normally rotate posteriorly with palpable lowering of posterior superior iliac spine on hip flexion.

Piriformis syndrome - Inflammation or spasm of the piriformis can cause sciatic nerve irritation because of their anatomic relationship. The sciatic nerve primarily runs below (87%) the piriformis muscle, although it may run through (12%) or above (<1%) the piriformis muscle in some cases. To reproduce piriformis muscle mediated pain, palpate the muscle between the lateral sacral edge and the greater trochanter; the sciatic nerve can be palpated midway between the ischial tuberosity and the greater trochanter with the hip in a flexed position. Piriformis syndrome can also be associated with leg length discrepancy and greater trochanteric bursitis. *Freiberg's test* produces buttock pain with forceful internal rotation of the flexed thigh. *Pace's maneuver* elicits pain by resisted hip abduction in the seated position. *Beatty's maneuver* produces pain by abducting/ externally rotating the flexed hip while side-lying with the affected side up (Beatty, 1994).

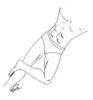

Figure 5d   Patrick's test.

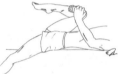

Figure 5e   Gaenslen's test.

Spondylolysis - If the spondylolysis is acute/ongoing, aggressive bracing (to prevent lumbar hyperextension) and a longer period of ongoing rest (hold lifting) should be considered in order to allow for pars healing or at least fibrous union. If the bone scan is negative (the spondylolysis is old or chronic), less aggressive lumbar bracing and a more expedient progression to spinal muscle strengthening could be considered.

Cauda equina syndrome - Signs of cauda equina syndrome such as urinary retention, bowel incontinence, saddle anesthesia (numbness in the sacral dermatomes), or erectile dysfunction necessitate urgent medical/surgical attention.

Pain amplification and suboptimal effort:

Hoover's test is used to gauge patient effort during an exam. With the patient laying supine and the examiner holding each heel, the patient is instructed to raise one leg. Effort to raise the leg should result in a downward force in the opposite leg. Lack of a downward force in the opposite leg implies a suboptimal lifting effort.

Waddell signs are signs suggestive of a non-organic basis for low back pain (LBP), e.g., malingering, psychiatric pathology in back pain patients, and are especially sensitive in chronic back pain. If 3 or more out of 5 signs are positive, a non-organic basis for low back pain (LBP), e.g., psychiatric problems, may be suspected. The five signs include:

1) *regionalization* - regional weakness/sensory loss in non-dermatomal pattern;
2) *overreaction* - exaggerated pain response to non-painful stimulus;
3) *simulation* - pain in the low back during manuevers not expected to stress the low back (e.g., placement of an axial loading force on the top of the head while standing or pain during sham rotation of the spine [i.e., the patient stands with feet together and the shoulders and hips are rotated together]);
4) *tenderness* - to superficial palpation; and
5) *distraction* - inconsistent findings during distraction, e.g., inconsistent pain response on sitting vs. supine SLR.

Gaines (1999) reported that patients with acute occupational LBP exhibiting at least one Waddell sign had a 4-fold lengthier time for return to unrestricted regular work and greater use of medical resources than patients without any Waddell signs.

Ref: Rubinstein SM, et al. A systematic review of the diagnostic accuracy of provocative tests of the neck for diagnosing cervical radiculopathy. *Eur J Spine* 2007;16:307.; **Malanga GA, et al.** Provocative tests in cervical spine examination: historical basis and scientific analyses. *Pain Physician* 2003;6:199; **Viikari-Juntura E, et al.** Validity of clinical tests in the diagnosis of root compression in cervical disc disease. *Spine* 1989;14:253; **van den Hoogen HM, et al.** On the accuracy of hx, PE, and ESR in diagnosing LBP in general practice. A criteria-based rev. of the lit. *Spine* 1995;20:318; **Vroomen PC, et al.** Diagnostic value of H&P in patients suspected of sciatica due to disc herniation: a systematic review. *J Neurol* 1999;246:899; **Waddell G, et al.** Nonorganic physical signs in LBP. *Spine* 1980;5:117; **Gaines WG, et al.** Effectiveness of Waddell's nonorganic signs in predicting a delayed return to regular work in patients experiencing acute occupational LBP. *Spine* 1999;24:396. **Figure credits: 5a, 5b, 5d, 5e.** Courtesy of **Dr. Jeffrey Ho**, with permission; **5c.** Courtesy of **Loeser JD, et al.**, eds. *Bonica's Management of Pain*, 3rd ed. Philadelphia, LWW, 2001, with permission.

Ch.6: ROLE OF LAB TESTS AND IMAGING IN THE EVALUATION OF PAIN

Labs - Serum chemistries, liver function tests, coagulation profiles, and complete blood counts not only may be necessary in the diagnosis of pathology, but are also important to ensure that patients will be able to metabolize drugs a pain medicine practitioner prescribes and safely tolerate invasive interventions that are offered. High rates of over-the-counter acetaminophen and NSAID use in some patients may warrant periodic checks of hepatic and renal function. Urine toxicology can be used to screen for illicit substance abuse and drug diversion.

Imaging - A specific differential diagnosis prior to ordering imaging is always suggested. Indiscriminate test ordering increases the likelihood of false positive findings, resulting in diagnostic confusion.

Plain films - The radiographic approach varies depending on the body region involved and the acuity/chronicity of pain. In chronic neck pain, with or without a history of trauma, an initial 3-view (AP, lateral, open mouth) radiographic series is recommended by the American College of Radiology (Daffner, 2005). Obliques can be ordered at the discretion of the physician. In acute neck pain due to trauma, high speed CT scanning has begun to replace plain films as the initial imaging modality of choice.

Uncomplicated acute low back pain does not warrant imaging studies according to the American College of Radiology (Bradley, 2005) and others. Although plain films are inexpensive and readily available, they can identify many abnormalities not related to symptoms. Abnormalities (e.g., spondylolysis, zygapophysial joint abnormalities, Schmorl's nodes, and mild scoliosis) can be equally prevalent in symptomatic and asymptomatic patients (Jarvik, 2002). In young females, it also needs to be considered that a single set of plain films of the lumbar spine results in gonadal radiation that is the equivalent of daily chest x-rays for several years (Jarvik, 2002).

Radiographs, as well as other tests, are indicated for back pain in the presence of "red flags" including: recent significant trauma (or milder trauma for age >50), unexplained weight loss, unexplained fever, immunosuppression, history of cancer, IV drug use, prolonged corticosteroid use, osteoporosis, age >70, focal neurologic deficit with progressive or disabling symptoms, or duration greater than 6 weeks (Bradley, 2005). Because pathology due to osteomyelitis or metastases may need to be fairly advanced before detection on plain radiography is likely, suspicion for these pathologic processes usually requires follow up with more advanced imaging modalities.

Standard film sets should include AP and lateral views. Oblique views of the lumbar spine (also known as the "Scottie dog" view) are useful in diagnosing spondylolysis if a pars interarticularis fracture (which corresponds to the "neck" of the Scottie dog) is suspected. Routine oblique views of the lumbar spine, however, are not supported by the literature (Jarvik, 2002). Flexion/extension views may be helpful to rule out unstable spondylolisthesis.

Computed tomography - CT is the imaging modality of choice to examine bony and calcific detail. Examples of indications where CT is superior to MRI include suspected fractures of the posterior elements of the spine and suspected ossification of the posterior longitudinal ligament. The postsurgical spine is also best imaged by CT due to the severe artifacts that can degrade MR images.

CT provides passable, if unexceptional, visualization of the soft tissues, for which modern MRI is generally superior. For instance, CTs are generally less useful in the examination of disc protrusions than MRI. CT also depicts the foraminal and extraforaminal nerve root fairly accurately due to the contrast provided by the surrounding fat, but is incapable of demonstrating the intrathecal nerve root or spinal cord without myelographic contrast (Jarvik, 2002). Myelography, when combined with CT, can outline the spinal cord, nerve roots and neural foraminae. It is the imaging modality of choice in examining patients with suspected radiculopathy who cannot tolerate MRI. CT myelogram is, in fact, considered by some to be the best test available for examining neuroforaminal anatomy, even superior to MRI, although it is not always clear how it will affect management. Even if it is assumed that the radiculopathy is due to compromise at the neural foramen, management may not change if ongoing conservative care is the appropriate management. Myelography also carries the risk of a potentially fatal anaphylactic reaction to the contrast, as well as the risk of infection and post-lumbar puncture headache.

Magnetic resonance imaging - MRI is the imaging modality of choice in examining the CNS parenchyma, as well as other soft tissues, including the spinal disc elements (annulus fibrosus, nucleus pulposus). Although MRIs do not directly visualize cortical bone, they can be useful in determining the acuity of fractures since the marrow edema and hematoma associated with acute fractures can be visualized.

T1-weighted images illustrate anatomic detail and are well suited for localization of masses and demonstration of mass effect on adjacent structures. T2-weighted images, although less anatomically detailed than T1-weighted images, provide information on many disease processes, such as infection, neoplasm, infarction, and white matter disease. Gadolinium, a paramagnetic contrast agent, has significantly increased the sensitivity and specificity of MRI, and is particularly useful for suspected infection or neoplasm. Enhancing tissues will appear bright on T1-weighted contrast enhanced images. Notably, gadolinium-containing contrast agents contain no iodine (i.e., they are safe in patients with iodine contrast allergy) and are not nephrotoxic (i.e., they can be used in patients with renal failure).

MRIs, on the other hand, also reveal many findings in persons who are asymptomatic (false-positives). Per Jensen (1994), 28% of asymptomatic population had at least one lumbar disc level with protrusion or extrusion. "High-intensity zones," for instance, refer to increased signals noted in the posterior annulus fibrosus, generally thought to represent tears. The clinical significance of these zones is equivocal, however, given the high prevalence of these zones in asymptomatic persons (Jarvik, 2002). Additionally, disc bulges and protrusions are common in asymptomatic persons, although disc extrusions (when noted to consist of extruded material with a narrower neck and broader distal element) are rare (1%; Jarvik 2002).

There are no known health risks associated with MRI. Contraindications include pacemakers, recent coronary bypass surgery (<24 hrs), spinal cord stimulators, ferromagnetic cerebral aneurysm clips, cochlear implants, and metallic foreign bodies in or around the orbits. Relative contraindications include external fixation devices and intrathecal pumps (can cause thermal burns).

Musculoskeletal ultrasound - has several advantages over other imaging techniques, including the lack of ionizing radiation and ability to perform a rapid real-time, dynamic study with the patient remaining in the examination room. Common applications include the imaging of suspected rotator cuff tears, Achilles tendon tears, muscle tears, and fluid collections in the joints and bursae. The procedure is also helpful in guiding the injection of medications into the sheaths around tendons. Musculoskeletal ultrasound is a promising and rapidly evolving modality.

Electrodiagnostics - can help to localize lesions and provide insight regarding the chronicity of pathology.

A common indication for a electrodiagnostic (EDx) testing referral is for the detection or ruling out of radiculopathy. Sensory and motor nerve conduction studies are usually normal in radiculopathy, although the motor results can be affected in severe cases. In the first 5–7 days, electromyography may demonstrate positive sharp waves and fibrillations (which are due to spontaneously contracting muscles secondary to denervation) in the paraspinal muscles, followed by similar findings in the distal musculature in a myotomal distribution at around 3–6 weeks post-injury. Although radiculopathy should not be ruled out within the first 4 weeks after a reported injury, demonstration of membrane instability within the first week or two post-injury may signify the presence of a prior pathological process. Eventually, denervation potentials due to radiculopathy may disappear with reinnervation, although reinnervation can require up to 2 yrs for the more distal muscles. Notably, a generalized presence of pathological waveforms (not in root distributions) can be normal in some persons.

EDx has several limitations with regards to the diagnosis of radiculopathy. EMG has a high specificity but lower sensitivity. In addition, there is a potential dearth of EDx findings in cases of radiculopathies involving dorsal root only.

EDx can also provide clues as to whether there might be secondary gain factors at play. Interference patterns on electromyography during voluntary contraction, for instance, can be decreased in patients who willfully do not provide maximal effort. On the other hand, a pattern of pathological waveforms, such as positive sharp waves in muscles innervated by the same root level correlating with a diagnosis of radiculopathy, cannot be produced voluntarily by persons seeking secondary gain.

Diagnostic injections for spinal pain - include provocation discography and diagnostic differential blocks. These tests are somewhat controversial, but can potentially aid in the demonstration of a pain generator, as well as its localization, when the other objective evidence is equivocal.

In the diagnostic differential block, a needle is placed into the area of interest, e.g., into the epidural or subdural space. A placebo, followed by increasing strengths of an anesthetic are injected. The patient is asked to state if there is pain relief following each of the injections. Pain relief after placebo injection is thought to be indicative of psychogenic pain. Lack of pain relief despite high concentration blockade, which is meant to block all sensory and sympathetic transmissions, may be indicative of central pain, encephalization of pain, or malingering. The epidural blockade has the advantage of not potentially causing the headache sometimes associated with the spinal, but requires more time to allow for the blockade to occur after each injection. Additional techniques for blockade of the stellate ganglion, brachial plexus, and lumbar paravertebral sympathetic chain exist. A successful diagnostic blockade, however, does not have a significant predictive value in terms of how well the "permanent" blockade might work (Raj, 1996).

Ref: Resnick, D. Bone and joint imaging. Philadelphia, WB Saunders, 1989; **Berquist TH.** MRI of the musculoskeletal system, 2nd ed. New York, Raven Press, 1990; **Bradley WG, et al.** Expert panel on neurologic imaging. Low Back Pain [online publication, AHRQ]. Reston (VA), Amer Coll of Radiology, 2005; **Freed JH, et al.** The use of the three-phase bone scan in the early diagnosis of heterotopic ossification (HO) and in the evaluation of Didronel therapy. *Paraplegia*. 1982;20:208; **Kaplan FS, et al.** Heterotopic ossification. *J Am Acad Orthop Surg*, 2004;12:116; **Daffner RH, et al.** Expert panel on musculoskeletal imaging. Chronic neck pain. [online publication, AHRQ]. Reston (VA), Amer Coll of Radiology, 2005; **Jarvik JG, Deyo RA.** Diagnostic evaluation of LBP w/ emphasis on imaging. *Ann Intern Med* 2002;137:586; **Jensen MC, et al.** Magnetic Resonance Imaging of the Lumbar Spine in People without Back Pain. *NEJM* 1994;331:69. **Raj PP.** *Pain medicine: A comprehensive review.* Mosby-Year Book, 1996.

Provocation discography

Discogenic pain - The outer third of the annulus fibrosus of the intervertebral disc contains neural fibers that are sensitive to chemical irritants from the nucleus pulposus, direct injury of annular fibers, and mechanical loads on the disc. Irritation of these fibers results in a predominantly axial neck or back pain. With lumbar discogenic pain, patients may experience discomfort in any position and often complain of pain that worsens with prolonged sitting, exercise, coughing, or sneezing. Discomfort

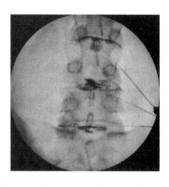

tends to be greatest in the lower back, but a significant amount of pain can also be experienced in the buttocks or lower extremities. Cervical discogenic pain typically involves the lower cervical discs and generally is not as disabling as lumbar discogenic pain. Symptoms typically are worsened with prolonged sitting, especially with the neck in flexion.

The role of discography - Discography is used to establish whether spinal pain is truly discogenic in nature. Injection of a pain-generating disc with saline and contrast dye is expected to reproduce pain, while injection of a healthy disc is not expected to result in pain. Pain induced by discography is thought to be secondary to: 1) increased disc pressure causing pressure on the annular fibers and/or vertebral end plates; and/or 2) chemical irritation of the pain-sensitive disc tissues.

For patients with normal or minimal findings on imaging, discography can establish an anatomical diagnosis. Annular tears, for instance, may not be apparent on MRI. For patients with abnormal findings on imaging, discography can confirm that the suspected disc is in fact the source of a patient's pain or demonstrate that it is not the pain generator (a large percentage of people with no spinal pain have disc abnormalities on MRI). Additionally, discography can also quantify the amount of pain from each disc tested. Specifically, establishing the affected disc levels helps to guide further treatment, which can include intradiscal electrothermic annuloplasty (IDEA) or surgery. Treatment can be tailored precisely to the affected levels and unnecessary interventions avoided (e.g., limiting a surgical fusion to 1 level instead of 2).

Specific indications for discography - The North American Spine Society clinical guidelines recommend that discography be considered in patients suffering from unremitting spinal pain without a definitive diagnosis despite adequate workup who have not responded to conservative treatments such as physical therapy, anti-inflammatory medications, muscle relaxants, or targeted spinal injections. Patients should have history, exam, and imaging findings consistent with potential discogenic pain and be prepared to proceed with further invasive therapy, such as IDEA or surgery. If discography is not anticipated to affect treatment decisions, the procedure should not be pursued.

Improving the reliability of discography - The key indicator of a positive test is reproduction of the patient's symptoms with injection of the disc or discs that are the pain generators. The reproduction of this pain, however, can be variable, and can depend on the pathology of the disc disorder, discographic technique, or psychological variables. Disc degeneration, for instance, is less likely to demonstrate a concordant pain on discography than for annular tears. Improper discographic techniques such as injecting the annular fibers or injecting too near the vertebral end plates can result in false positive results. Finally, patients with certain psychological variables frequently have false positive discograms. Therefore, psychological status clearance prior to discography is recommended (Carragee, 2000), although a formal psych consult is not always necessarily required. Injections of adjacent "control" discs and sham injections have been proposed as methods to improve the reliability of discography. It should be noted, however, that even injection of a so-called normal or healthy disc can result in increased pressure that can in turn lead to pain.

    Contraindications - include increased risk of bleeding due to coagulopathy or medications (aspirin, clopidogrel, ticlopidine, warfarin, NSAIDs), immunocompromised states, systemic or local skin infections, and significant underlying psychopathology. Discography should not be pursued if fluoroscopy cannot be utilized or if the patient is unable to lie still.

Discography procedure

- Anxiolytics or sedatives may be used. The patient, however, must be awake, alert, capable of conveying symptoms, and be able to converse for the test to be valid.
- The skin is prepped thoroughly (discitis can result if the patient's skin is inadequately cleansed).
- Local anesthetic is injected into the entry site on the skin.
- Cranial/caudal tilt and oblique angulation is used to best visualize a path into the disc. A large bore needle is directed under fluoroscopic guidance towards the disc. This is repeated for each disc level to be studied.
- A "double needle" technique using a second smaller gauge needle that goes through the first needle may be used to deliver the injectate into the disc. The double needle technique reduces the chance of discitis.
- Nonionic contrast (with or without antibiotics, e.g., cefazolin) is injected into the nucleus pulposus, while carefully monitoring the flow pattern (e.g., the presence of fissures or herniations) and patient response (e.g., pressure sensations and numeric rating scales for pain).
- If pain is provoked and is concordant with the usual symptoms, the disc is noted to be a pain generator; the volume of injectate that elicited pain reproduction should be recorded.
- Post-discography CT scanning is frequently ordered. It can be helpful in the planning of future procedures.
- Ice and analgesics may mitigate post-procedural pain.

Risks and complications of discography - Post-procedural pain is common, although the discomfort is typically short-lived (~1–2 days). Discitis is a rare but major complicaton that is difficult to treat due to poor intradiscal blood supply. Its incidence is theoretically minimized by mixing antibiotics with the contrast media, although this is not a universally accepted practice, especially with the double needle technique, which by itself has resulted in decreased infection rates (Willems, 2004). Other complications include: vasovagal reaction; allergic reaction to the contrast, nerve root injury or radiculitis, thecal sac puncture (more likely with transdural approaches), and epidural hemorrhage or abscess (very unlikely). Cerebral vascular accidents secondary to particulate from the steroids entering the vasculature following a cervical discography have been reported.

Ref: Carragee EJ, et al. The rates of false-positive lumbar discography in select patients w/o low back symptoms. *Spine* 2000;25:1373; **Willems PC, et al**. Lumbar discography: should we use prophylactic antibiotics? A study of 435 consecutive discograms and a systematic review of the literature. *J Spinal Disord Tech* 2004;17:243. **Figure credit:** Radiograph courtesy of **Ballantyne JC**. *The MGH Handbook of Pain Management*, 3rd ed. Philadelphia, LWW, 2006, with permission.

Ch.7: PSYCHOLOGICAL AND FUNCTIONAL EVALUATION

Pain and psychological function are initimately linked. Depression is thought to be highly prevalent in patients with chronic pain, and Currie (2004) showed that severity of pain correlated with the rate of major depression. Treatment outcomes in pain management, e.g., spine surgery, have been shown to be predictable by psychological evaluation.

The psychological evaluation consists of a clinical interview, mental status exam, pain screening inventories or pain scales (e.g., visual analog scale, McGill Pain Questionnaire), psychiatric screening or standardized testing, and measures of psychological and behavioral function.

Screening psychiatric testing - examples include the Beck Depression Inventory (BDI) and Symptom Checklist-90-R (SCL-90-R). Many screens, including BDI and SCL-90-R, have high levels of face-validity, meaning that the tests are easily manipulated by patients who seek to misrepresent their emotional state.

The **Beck Depression Inventory** (Beck and Steer, 1987) is a 21 item, 10 min depression screen. Scores of 0–9 correlate with no depression, whereas score above 30 suggests severe depression. A positive screen requires diagnostic confirmation. The **Symptom Checklist-90-R** examines psychological symptoms, takes about 15 mins to complete, and is often used on patient intake. Patients screening positively are followed up with a Minnesota Multiphasic Personality Inventory (MMPI-2). SCL-90-R can also be used to monitor progress during treatment.

Standardized psychiatric testing - examples include the MMPI-2 and Millon Clinical Multiaxial Inventory III.

The **Minnesota Multiphasic Personality Inventory (MMPI-2)** is a 1989 revision of the original MMPI scale developed in the 1930s at University of Minnesota. It is considered a "gold standard" for describing personality or psychological disorders, although it should not be used alone for a diagnosis, and test results are often misinterpreted by non-experts. The long form contains 567 true-false questions which ordinarily takes about 2 hrs to complete, although patients with severe or chronic pain can take several sessions to finish the test. In pain medicine, the MMPI-2 is used to assess patients, help tailor treatment strategies, and predict response to treatment and outcomes, although the latter must be done with caution. Psychopathology disorders noted during the acute pain stage were traditionally thought to be predictors for chronic pain, although more recent research is less supportive of this. The MMPI-2 has low face validity; manipulating the test to misrepresent psychological states can be detected. **The Millon Clinical Multiaxial Inventory III** is shorter than the MMPI-2 and correlates with DSM-IV diagnoses.

The **Millon Behavioral Medicine Diagnostic** is a test for personality which is unique in that it has been standardized on medical patients. It is useful to assess how a patient is coping with the stress of physical illness, including pain. For patients being considered for invasive medical therapies, this test has specific scales which measure the patient's emotional reaction to such planned treatments.

Functional scales are commonly used scales to follow function during chronic pain treatment and include the 36-Item Short Form Health Survey (Short Form 36 or SF-36), Multidimensional Pain Inventory (MPI), Oswestry Disability Index (ODI), and Barthel Index.

The **36-Item Short Form Health Survey (SF-36)** was developed by the RAND Corp. as part of the multi-site Medical Outcomes Study to explain variability in patient outcomes. It is a widely used quality of life survey not targeted for a specific disease. It is useful in surveys of populations, comparing the relative burden of diseases and benefits of various treatments. The SF-12 is a 2-minute variation that has been shown to achieve the minimum standards of validity.

The ***Multidimensional Pain Inventory (MPI)*** focuses on behavioral factors to evaluate the ability to cope with pain. Patients are categorized as either dysfunctional, interpersonally distressed, or as an adaptive coper.

The ***Oswestry Disability Index (ODI)*** takes about 10 mins to complete. ODI questionnaire was first published in 1980. Some consider it the "gold standard" for low back functional outcomes, but it has not been validated in other conditions. There are 10 items on nine aspects of daily living and pain medication use. A modified version, ***Neck Disability Index***, has been described for neck pain.

The ***Barthel Index*** reports the degree of disability. The goal is to establish any degree of independence from help, physical or verbal. It is principally concerned with physical aspects of disability, emphasizing what a subject does, not could do. It is best when recorded over periods of time by a single individual. A score of 14 (out of 20) indicates some disability, but is usually compatible with the level of support found in a residential home. A score of 10 is compatible with discharge home provided there is a caregiver present.

Ref: Ware JE, Sherbourne CD. The MOS 36-item short-form health survey (SF-36): I. Conceptual framework and item selection. *Medical Care* 1992;30:473; **Currie SR, Wang J**. Chronic back pain and major depression in the general Canadian population. *Pain* 2004;107:54.

Part Two
Treatment Modalities

Ch.8: GOALS OF TREATMENT; MULTIDISCIPLINARY CARE; DISABILITY

The goal of treatment is to: 1) eliminate pain when possible; or to 2) manage pain and restore function when eliminating the pain is not possible. Typical first-line treatments include rehabilitation, pharmacological analgesics, adjuvant therapies, and alternative/complementary treatments. Psychological therapies, surgical/anesthetic techniques, and a formal multidisciplinary approach may be necessary in select cases. Pain physicians are also frequently requested to comment on and certify disability.

The multidisciplinary approach - Given the varied impairments in the physical, psychological, social, and vocational domains due to pain, a multidisciplinary approach to management is frequently advocated for and has been generally supported by the peer-reviewed literature, although the quality of the supportive literature has not typically been high-grade. In 1992, Flor, et al., published a metanalysis of 56 studies showing an advantage of multidisciplinary care in terms of pain control, return to work, and healthcare utilization over individual treatment with medication management or physical therapy alone. The authors stated, however, that the quality of the study designs reviewed was "marginal" and that further research was necessary.

More recent literature has improved in design quality but has shown somewhat equivocal results. A 2005 Swedish study (Jensen) showed benefits and cost-effectiveness of a multidisciplinary program over less intensive options for women but not men in regards to sick leave, early retirement, and health-related quality of life during a 3 year follow up period of patients identified during sick leave for neck and back pain. McAllister, et al., (2005) showed that a 4 wk mutlidisciplinary program was effective in improving pain ratings, opioid use, healthcare utilization, and perceived physical function for up to 12 mos after program discharge in patients with refractory chronic pain. Kaapa, et al., (2006) showed that in patients with chronic non-specific back pain, a 70 hr semi-intensive multidisciplinary program did not show marginal benefit with regards to pain scores and disability over a 10 hr individual physiotherapy program by practitioners using a cognitive-behavioral approach. More research is clearly indicated.

Disability - Despite treatment, patients with pain may not have enough function restored to perform ADLs or return to work. Systems for healthcare and financial support during this phase include workers' compensation and Social Security Disability.

Workers' compensation covers employees injured due to work. Employers cover the costs of insurance; employees, in turn, relinquish the right to hold employers liable for injuries. While the rules vary by state, typical employee benefits include coverage of medical care, vocational rehabilitation, and temporary and permanent disability payments. Medical costs have historically been lower than disability payments, incentivizing insurers to seek expedient and optimal functional recovery rather than to minimize medical costs per se. Programs to improve function such as work hardening which are also generally supported by the medical literature (Schonstein, 2002) are often utilized.

Impairments are determined using state-specific guidelines, often based on the *AMA's Guide to the Evaluation of Permanent Impairment*. Generally, pain can only add up to 3% to the whole person impairment when another impairment has been demonstrated. Disability is determined by the legal system.

Social Security Disability (SSD) in the United States is a federal program that pays a benefit for people who can no longer work because of a medical condition expected to last ≥1 yr or result in death. Physicians and disability specialists evaluate each application for functional impairments. For SSD, pain, in the absence of objective signs or abnormal test results, is not considered an impairment (and w/o impairments disability cannot be established). Moreover, if it is deemed that the applicant can perform any other work (e.g., sedentary work), the agency will decide that there is no disability. The applicant's personal physicians are not asked to decide whether the applicant is disabled.

Ref: Flor H, et al. Efficacy of multidisciplinary pain treatment centers: a meta-analytic review. *Pain* 1992;49:221; **Jensen IB, et al**. A 3-year follow-up of a multidisciplinary rehabilitation programme for back and neck pain. *Pain* 2005;115:273; **McAllister MJ, et al**. Effectiveness of a multidisciplinary chronic pain program for treatment of refractory patients with complicated chronic pain syndromes. *Pain Physician* 2005;8:369; **Kaapa EH, et al**. Multidisciplinary group rehabilitation versus individual physiotherapy for chronic nonspecific LBP: a randomized trial. *Spine* 2006;15:371; **Schonstein E, et al**. Work conditioning, work hardening and functional restoration for workers with back and neck pain. *Cochrane Database System Rev* 2002;4:CD001822.

Ch.9: REHABILITATION IN PAIN MANAGEMENT

Pain can be exacerbated by ongoing injury, disuse of affected body parts, general deconditioning, and disability. Physical medicine and rehabilitation (PM&R) interventions aim to directly address these issues, complementing and reinforcing pharmacological and psychological treatments.

Despite empiric support for these modalities, however, there is little high-grade experimental evidence demonstrating objective benefits. The oft-cited *Philadelphia Panel Physical Therapy* study, for instance, found little or no supporting evidence to use the following modalities for the treatment of acute (<6 wks) low back pain: mechanical traction, therapeutic exercise, massage, ultasound, TENS, EMG biofeedback, and postural re-education. Nonetheless, the use of selected PM&R modalities is clearly warranted in cases involving motivated patients, where the emphasis is placed on functional recovery (i.e., of ADLs or return to work) and functional status is closely monitored.

Orthoses - *Back brace (back support)*: a prospective cohort study over 2 years involving thousands of material-handling employees in 30 states revealed that neither frequent back braces use nor policies requiring back brace use were associated with reduced incidence of back injury claims or low back pain (Wassell, 2000). Other studies have also failed to demonstrate the utility of lumbar supports, corsets, braces, or other orthoses in preventing back pain or injury.

Manual therapy - involves a "hands-on" approach and includes modalities such as massage, soft tissue mobilization, and manipulation. *Massage* is the stroking, friction, and kneading of muscles and soft tissues. Stroking maneuvers can decrease edema and produce muscle relaxation. Friction and kneading massage break down intramuscular adhesions and prepare the muscles and soft tissues for stretching. *Myofascial release* is a method of soft tissue mobilization that focuses on the fascial component believed to cause pain and dysfunction.

Manipulation is a skilled, passive movement of a spinal segment, usually within and occasionally beyond its active range of motion. Various professionals, including osteopathic physicians, chiropractors, and primary care physicians, use spinal manipulation but differ in the rationale and techniques used.

When combined with exercise, mobilization and manipulation techniques have been shown to be effective for subacute and chronic mechanical neck disorders with or without headache (Gross, 2004). Mobilization or manipulation alone, however, were not effective and there was insufficient literature to support either of these modalities in the presence of radicular pain.

The older evidence-based literature had generally been supportive, if somewhat lukewarmly, of manipulation techniques as primary or adjunctive therapies in nonspecific low back pain. A now classic study published in the *New England Journal of Medicine* (Cherkin, 1998) compared McKenzie-style physical therapy (PT), chiropractic manipulation, and educational booklet as treatments for patients with nonradiating low back pain. The study found that manipulation was at least as effective as PT. Both therapies were slightly superior to the booklet. A Cochrane Back Review Group review found that manipulative therapy had no clinical advantage over general practitioner care, analgesics, PT, or exercise therapy (Assendelft, 2003). A randomized sham-controlled trial conducted at the Texas Coll. of Osteopathic Med., however, showed benefit from both osteopathic and sham manipulation when used as adjunctive therapies to conventional care, making it unclear if the benefits were due to manipulation or time spent interacting with patients, representing placebo effects (Licciardone, 2003).

Traction involves the manual or mechanical distraction of vertebral bodies and facet joints to reduce pain from nerve irritation. The current literature does not support or refute the effectiveness of traction for neck pain when compared to placebo traction or other treatment modalities (Graham, 2008). Lumbar traction is not supported by the evidence-based medical literature (Clarke, 2006).

Ref: Philadelphia Panel. Evidence-based clinical practice guidelines on selected rehab. interventions for LBP. *Physical Therapy* 2001;81:1641; **Wassell JT, et al**. A prospective study of back belts for prevention of back pain and injury. *JAMA* 2000;284:2727; **Gross AR, et al**. Manipulation and mobilisation for mechanical neck disorders. *Cochrane Database Syst Rev* 2004;(1):CD004249; **Cherkin DC, et al**. A comparison of PT, chiropractic manip., and provision of an educational booklet for the tx of pts with LBP. *N Engl J Med* 1998;339:1021; **Assendelft WJ, et al**. Spinal manip. tx for LBP. A metanalysis of effectiveness relative to other txs. *Ann Intern Med* 2003;138:871; **Licciardone JC, et al**. Osteopathic manipulative tx for chronic LBP: a RCT. *Spine* 2003;28:1355; **Graham N, et al**. Mechanical traction for neck pain with or without radiculopathy. *Cochrane Database Syst Rev* 2008;(3):CD006408; **Clarke J, et al**. Traction for LBP w/ or w/o sciatica: an updated systematic review w/in the framework of the Cochrane collaboration. *Spine* 2006;31:1591.

Exercise - *Therapeutic exercise* is designed to increase functional activity. Exercises include range of motion, stretching, strengthening, general cardiovascular conditioning, and relaxation exercises.

Stretching should include muscles that cross two joints such as the hamstrings, gastrocsoleous group, hip flexors, pectorals, finger flexors and extensors, and paraspinal muscles. Some of these muscles frequently become tight and shortened, causing poor posture and pain.

Strengthening exercises include: isotonic exercises, where there is active contraction of muscle against resistance with movement; and isometric exercises, where the muscle length is unchanged but tension is increased. Isometric exercises are often thought to be the safest during the early stages when injured joints or bones are still healing. For spinal strengthening, the Williams flexion exercises generally recommended in the 1950s were replaced by McKenzie extension exercises in the 1980s, and then by combined lumbar stabilization exercises in the 1990s.

Relaxation exercises reduce anxiety, autonomic hyperactivity, and muscle tension, all seen in chronic pain states. Techniques such as imagery, progressive muscle relaxation, controlled breathing, or listening to relaxation tapes are commonly used to manage chronic pain.

Exercise therapy programs have been shown to be slightly effective at decreasing pain and improving function in adults with chronic low back pain (Hayden, 2005). In subacute low back pain, graded exercise activity programs improve absentee outcomes, while in acute back pain, exercise therapy shows no advantage over no therapy or other conservative treatments (Hayden, 2005).

Ref: Hayden JA, et al. Exercise therapy for treatment of non-specific low back pain. *Cochrane Database Syst Rev* 2005;(3):CD000335.

Thermal modalities - Analgesia produced by heat can be explained by the gate-control theory of pain modulation. Heat increases blood flow, presumably leading to the acceleration of healing. Heat can also increase flexibility of collagenous tissues, which may be helpful before stretching. In patients with adhesive capsulitis ("frozen shoulder") or postsurgical scarring, for instance, ultrasound followed by deep massage and stretching can be effective.

Superficial heat elevates the temperature of tissues and provides the greatest effect at <0.5 cm from the surface of the skin. Fluidotherapy circulates warm air through small cellulose granules under thermostatic control. An advantage of fluidotherapy over hydrotherapy is decreased edema due to a decreased reliance on dependent positions.

Deep heating (diathermy) increases temperature to depths of 3–5 cm by converting other forms of energy to heat. Examples include shortwave diathermy (high-frequency electrical currents), microwave diathermy (electromagnetic radiation), and ultrasound (high-frequency acoustic vibrations). Ultrasound is a preferred treatment in most painful disorders due to its excellent penetration and its safety around metal. It also increases the extensibility of tissue and thus is helpful in treating trigger points, tight tendons, and capsular structures.

Contraindications to heat include treatment of areas with active malignancy. Microwave and shortwave diathermy techniques are contraindicated in the presence of metal and pacemakers, because metals selectively absorb energy and generate heat that can damage surrounding tissues. Microwave diathermy also selectively heats tissue with high water content and thus is contraindicated over joints with effusions or cavities with fluids.

Cryotherapy *(the application of cold)* is the immediate treatment of choice after acute injuries. It is also frequently used on trigger points after a muscle is injected. Cryotherapy reduces the metabolic activity of underlying tissues, slows nerve conduction and, by its direct effect on muscle spindle activity, reduces muscle spasm and guarding. Anectodal evidence suggests that cold therapy may be more effective in muscle pain than heat.

Electrotherapy - has been used since ancient times when "torpedo fish" that produced electric currents were used to treat gout and headaches.

Transcutaneous electrical nerve stimulation (TENS) is the delivery of electrical energy across the skin surface to stimulate the peripheral nervous system. The rationale for TENS is based on the gate-control theory of pain modulation. The typical TENS unit delivers variable amounts of current at variable pulse rates and durations. A biphasic waveform (no net DC current) is preferred to minimize the skin irritation (due to electrolytic effects) characteristic of a unidirectional current. TENS should not be used in patients with pacemakers and be used cautiously in patients with spinal cord stimulators or intrathecal pumps. TENS should be avoided during pregnancy due to the possibility of premature labor induction.

Conventional TENS settings include an amplitude just above sensory threshold, a high frequency (40–150 Hz), and short duration (10–50 μs). Pain relief typically only occurs during active treatment. "Acupuncture-like" TENS using higher amplitudes and lower frequencies and is said to result in longer duration pain relief (extending beyond active use of the TENS device), but is not tolerated by some patients.

Although TENS has widespread applications, it is sometimes said to be most effective in the early stages of mild to moderate pain, especially neuropathic pain such as CRPS, phantom pain, and postherpetic neuralgia. A general consensus is that analgesia with TENS is often quite successful initially, but that persistent ongoing relief over the successive months to years is infrequent. Systematic reviews, particularly, have not demonstrated clear evidence of effect on chronic pain or functional amelioration in properly designed trials (Nnoaham, 2008; Khadilkar, 2005).

Nevertheless, despite the general lack of high-grade supportive medical literature, the closely monitored use of relatively inexpensive non-invasive palliative modalities such as TENS, particularly in non-chronic pain, is supported in clinical practice, provided that the emphasis is placed on functional restoration.

Inferential stimulation is a transcutaneous electrical stimulation modality using alternating current signals of different frequency. While there are theoretical advantages to using inferential stimulation patterns, clear clinical superiority over TENS has not been demonstrated. Likewise, high-grade medical literature supporting the use of inferential stimulators in chronic musculoskeletal conditions or chronic pain has yet to be published.

Percutaneous neuromodulation therapy or ***percutaneous electrical nerve stimulation (PENS)*** delivers electrical stimulation via percutaneous needle probes. While it is presumably advantageous to bypass skin resistance, PENS does require a visit to a practitioner. Pilot studies suggest some potential for short-term relief of pain, as well as potential for short-term subjective functional benefits. There is no data as yet supporting a sustained long-term functional or analgesic benefit for this modality.

Miscellaneous - ***EMG biofeedback*** uses surface EMG electrodes to provide a patient real-time visual or auditory feedback regarding muscle activity. The aim is to help patients learn to reduce their own muscle activity to reduce spasms and reduce pain.

Controlled trials establishing the clinical efficacy of biofeedback therapy, however, are lacking to date. In neck pain, the last published systematic search for trials was by Kjellman (1999), which demonstrated no qualifying trials. In chronic low back pain, a literature review showed no benefit of EMG biofeedback over placebo in pain control or function (van Tulder, 1997).

Low level laser therapy (LLLT) is a modality that is reported to increase circulation, resulting in biological healing and pain relief. LLLT causes only a minimal increase in local temperature, which is not felt to be responsible for the reported effects.

The literature on LLLT for pain syndromes is mixed. Basford, et al., (1999) found that treatment with low-intensity 1.06 micron laser irradiation produced a moderate reduction in pain and improvement in function in patients with musculoskeletal low back pain. Benefits, however, were limited and decreased with time. The authors concluded that further research was warranted. Bingol, et al., (2005) found no significant improvement in pain, active range, or algometric sensitivity in patients with shoulder pain treated with laser in comparison to controls. However, a metanalysis by Chow, et al., (2009) concluded that LLLT reduces pain immediately after treatment in acute neck pain and up to 22 weeks after completion of treatment in patients with chronic neck pain based on 16 randomized controlled trials (n = 820).

Ref: Nnoaham KE, Kumbang J. TENS for chronic pain. *Cochrane Database Syst Rev* 2008;(3):CD003222; **Khadilkar A, et al.** TENS for the treatment of chronic LBP: a systematic review. *Spine* 2005;30:2657; **Kjellman GV, et al.** A critical analysis of RCTs on neck pain and treatment efficacy. A review of the literature. *Scand J Rehabil Med* 1999;31:139; **van Tulder MW, et al.** Conservative treatment of acute and chronic nonspecific LBP. A systematic review of RCTs of the most common interventions. *Spine* 1997;22:2128; **Basford JR, et al.** Laser therapy: a randomized, controlled trial of the effects of low-intensity Nd:YAG laser irradiation on musculoskeletal back pain. *Arch Phys Med Rehab* 1999;80:647; **Bingol U, et al.** Low-power laser treatment for shoulder pain. *Photomed Laser Surg* 2005;23:459; **Chow RT, et al.** Efficacy of low-level laser therapy in the management of neck pain: a systemic review and meta-analysis of randomised placebo or active-treatment controlled trials. *Lancet* 2009; 374:1897.

Ch.10: COMMON NON-OPIOID PAIN MEDICATIONS

Notes: the following doses are for typical-sized adults. *Contraindications* always include hypersensitivity to the drug itself; "*Warn/Prec*" are warnings and precautions. "Most common" side effects may be marked with an asterisk. The information contained herein is abridged; please refer to the PDR or product inserts for more information.

Antidepressants

amitriptyline (Elavil, Merck) - [tabs 10, 25, 50, 75, 100, 150 mg] *Indic/ Dosage*: depression: 50–150 mg qhs (for elderly 10 mg tid and 20 mg qhs may be sufficient; reduce dose for hepatic impairment); off-label for neuropathic pain (start at doses lower than for depression); *Action*: tertiary amine tricyclic, NE/serotonin reuptake inhibitor; also has anti α1-adrenergic and potent antimuscarinic properties; Contra: acute post-MI, concomitant MAOI use; *Warn/Prec*: CV disorders (can cause HTN), hyperthyroidism, schizophrenia/ paranoia, pregnancy D, discontinue before elective surgery; withdraw gradually after long-term use to avoid insomnia and abdominal discomfort; black box warning for increased risk of suicidality in < 25 years old; *Adverse Rxs*: dry mouth*, blurred vision*, constipation*, urinary retention*, cardiovascular effects (tachycardia*, prolongation of AV conduction), drug fever, leukopenia, weight gain, somnolence, seizures, photosensitivity, rash, abdominal distress, gynecomastia, testicular swelling, menstrual irregularity, sexual dysfunction; *Monitoring*: baseline and periodic leukocyte and differential counts, LFTs, ECG; pts with cardiovascular issues require surveillance.

desipramine (Norpramin, Sanofi-Aventis) - [tabs 10, 25, 50, 75, 100, and 150 mg] *Indic/Dosage*: depression; off-label use includes treatment of neuropathic pain and ADHD. Start 25–100 mg qday or in divided doses. Usual effective dose is 100–200 mg/d, max 300 mg/d. *Action*: primarily inhibits norepinephrine reuptake; *Contra*: In the acute recovery phase after MI, concomitant MAOI use; *Adverse Rxs:* blurred vision, constipation, drowsiness. dry mouth or hypotension; *Monitoring*: pts with hx of cardiovascular disease require closer surveillance. Black box warning for increased risk of suicidality in those < 25 years old.

duloxetine (Cymbalta, Eli Lilly) - [delayed-release caps 20, 30, 60 mg] *Indic/ Dosage*: FDA-approved for depression (40–60 mg daily) and in 2003 for diabetic peripheral neuropathy; *Action*: selective serotonin and norepinephrine reuptake inhibitor; *Contra*: end-stage renal disease (requiring dialysis) or in severe renal impairment (estimated CrCl <30 mL/min); *Warn/Prec*: CV disorders (can cause HTN), hyperthyroidism, schizophrenia/paranoia, pregnancy C, d/c before elective surgery; withdraw gradually after long-term use to avoid insomnia and abdominal discomfort, drug interactions (with TCAs, phenothiazines, and type 1C antiarrhythmics) black box warning for increased risk of suicidality in those < 25 years old; *Adverse Rxs*: nausea*, somnolence*, dry mouth*, urinary hesitancy; *Monitoring*: BP and HR, check efficacy after 12 weeks, observe coexisting depression/bipolar disorder for suicide risk or mania/ hypomania.

milnacipran (Savella, Cypress Bioscience) - [tabs 12.5, 25, 50, 100 mg] *Indic/ Dosage*: FDA-approved for fibromyalgia; Off-label use for depression. Dosing should be titrated according to the following schedule: Day 1: 12.5 mg once, Days 2–3: 25 mg/day (12.5 mg twice daily), Days 4–7: 50 mg/day (25 mg twice daily), After Day 7: 100 mg/day (50 mg twice daily). Daily maximum 200 mg/day; *Action*: serotonin and norepinephrine reuptake inhibitor. *Warn/ Prec*: Not approved for pediatric patients. Black box warning for increased risk of suicidality in those < 25 years old, coadministration with a monoamine oxidase inhibitor (MAOI) or use within 14 days of initiating or discontinuing therapy with an MAOI is not recommended; caution in patients with hepatic and renal dysfunction; pregnancy C; *Adverse Rxs:* nausea*, palpitations*; dry mouth; headache; constipation; hyperhydrosis, vomiting, dizziness. *Monitoring*: BP and HR, depressive sx and suicide risk; withdrawal sx when discontinued; serotonin syndrome or neuroleptic malignant syndrome (NMS)-like reactions.

mirtazapine (Remeron, Organon) - [tabs 15, 30, 45 mg; orally disintegrating (SolTab) 15, 30, 45 mg] *Indic/Dosage:* FDA-approved for depression; Off-label use for anxiety and neuropathic pain; start 15 mg po qhs, titrate up to q 1–2 weeks to 45 mg/d; *Action:*Enhances central serotonergic and noradrenergic activity via activity as antagonist central presynaptic α2 adrenergic receptor; potent 5-HT2 and 5-HT3 receptor angatonist; potent histamine H1-receptor antagonist; moderate alpha-1 adrenergic antagonist; moderate muscarinic receptor antagonist; metabolized via CYP2D6 and 1As; *Warn/Prec*: Blackbox warning for increased risk of suicidality in children, adolescents and young adults; coadministration with a monoamine oxidase inhibitor (MAOI) or use within 14 days of initiating or discontinuing therapy with an MAOI is not recommended; caution in patients with hepatic and renal dysfunction; avoid Sol Tab in phenylketonurics (contains phenylalanine); pregnancy C; *Adverse Rxs:* Somnolence*, dizziness*, asthenia*, increased appetite/weight gain*, dry mouth*, constipation, nausea, hypercholesterolemia, ALT (SGPT) elevation, activation of hypomania/mania, seizure, rare agranulocytosis.

nortriptyline (Palemor, Mallinckrodt; Aventyl, Ranbaxy) - [caps 10, 25, 50, 75 mg. Oral solution 10 mg/5 ml] *Indic/Dosage*: depression; off-label use includes chronic pain modification (including temporomandibular joint disorder) and prevention of migraines. Start 25 mg qhs or divided bid-qid. Usual effective dose is 75–100 mg/d, max 150 mg/d. *Action*: primarily inhibits norepinephrine reuptake, and to a lesser extent serotonin; *Contra*: In the acute recovery phase after MI, concomitant MAOI use; *Adverse Rxs:* dry mouth, drowsiness, orthostatic hypotension, urinary retention, constipation, irregular heartbeat, and sexual dysfunction; *Monitoring*: pts with hx of cardiovascular disease, stroke, glaucoma, and/or seizures require closer surveillance. Obtain EKG at baseline and monitor for QT prolongation.

venlafaxine (Effexor, Pfizer) - [caps, extended release (Effexor XR) 37.5, 75, 150 mg; tabs 25, 37.5, 50, 75, 100 mg] *Indic/Dosage*: FDA-approved for depression, generalized anxiety disorder, social anxiety disorder and panic disorder; off-label use for neuropathic pain and migraine prophylaxis; start 25 mg po tid (or 75 mg/d if using Effexor XR), titrate every 4 days up to 225 mg/d; *Action*: selective serotonin and norepinephrine reuptake inhibitor; metabolized via CYP2D6; *Warn/Prec*: Blackbox warning for increased risk of suicidality in children, adolescents, and young adults; avoid co-administration with MAOI; avoid starting venlafaxine within 14 days of discontinuing MAOI; avoid starting MAOI until at least 7 days after discontinuing venlafaxine; monitor for serotonin syndrome if using venlafaxine together with SNRI, SSRI or triptans; may cause hypertension; may cause mydriasis, hence monitor those at risk for narrow-angle glaucoma; may lead to hyponatremia, bleeding; hypercholesterolemia, interstitial lung disease, eosinophilic pneumonia; pregnancy C; *Adverse Rxs:* abnormal ejaculation*, anorgasmia*, impotence*, somnolence*, dry mouth*, sweating*, nausea*, decreased libido*, abnormal dreams, nervousness, pharyngitis, constipation, flatulence, insomnia, tremor, abnormal vision, hypertension, vasodilation, yawning, anorexia; *Monitoring*: BP and HR; check for mania/hypomania; check efficacy after 12 weeks; monitor height and weight in pediatric patients; **desvenlafaxine** (Pristiq, Pfizer – [extended release tabs 50, 100 mg]) is metabolite of venlafaxine and is FDA-approved for major depressive disorder. Taken qd.

Spasticity/Muscle Hyperactivity

baclofen (Lioresal, Novartis) - [tabs 10, 20 mg; intrathecal] *Indic/Dosage*: spasticity: titrate to max dose of 20 mg qid as follows: 5 mg tid × 3d, then 10 mg tid × 3d, then 15 mg tid × 3d, then 20 mg tid × 3d, increase as needed; consider intrathetcal (IT) pump if oral route is effective but titration is limited by side-effects; no indication of oral form for spasticity due to stroke, Parkinson's disease, or cerebral palsy; *Action*: analog of γ-aminobutyric acid thought to bind to GABA-B receptors, inhibiting Ca influx into presynaptic terminals and suppressing spinal cord excitatory neurotransmitters; *Warn/Prec*: impaired renal fxn, risk of seizure if withdrawn too quickly (therefore, should taper off over approximately 1wk or so), pregnancy C; *Adverse Rxs* (oral baclofen): drowsiness*, dizziness*, headache*, N/V*, lassitude*, GI upset*, urinary frequency, confusion, CNS depression, slurred speech, seizures, blurred vision, nasal congestion, weakness, hypotonia, HTN, CV collapse, respiratory failure, pruritus, rash, increased LFTs; (IT baclofen): fatigue*, drowsiness*; *Overdosage*: IV physostigmine 1–2 mg.

clonidine (Catapres, Boehringer Ingelheim) - [tabs 0.1, 0.2, 0.3 mg; TTS qwk patch 0.1/24, 0.2/24, 0.3 mg/24 hr] *Indic/Dosage*: HTN: start orally at 0.1–0.3 mg bid, or TTS 0.1 mg/24 hr qwk, maximum dose is 2.4 mg/d orally or TTS 0.3 mg/24 hr qwk; off label for spasticity: dosing similar to HTN; IT clonidine used investigationally for spasticity and neuropathic pain; *Action*: central α-adrenergic agonist that ↓ sympathetic discharge; *Warn/Prec*: CV disease, impaired liver/renal fxn, withdraw gradually to avoid rebound HTN, pregnancy C; *Adverse Rxs*: dry mouth/eyes, h/a, dizziness, nausea, constipation, sedation, weakness, fatigue, orthostatic hypotension, edema, anorexia, erectile dysfunction, joint pain, leg cramps.

cyclobenzaprine (Flexeril, McNeil) - [tabs 5, 10 mg] *Indic/Dosage*: muscle spasm due to acute painful musculoskeletal conditions: 10 mg tid, max 60 mg/d, not to exceed 2-3 wks; *Action*: structurally related to the TCAs; thought to act on the brainstem to reduce skeletal muscle hyperactivity, but not effective for spasticity of central origin; *Contra*: TCA hypersensitivity, concomitant MAOIs (or w/in 14d of d/c), recovery from acute MI, CHF, arrhythmias, conduction disturbances, hyperthyroidism; *Warn/Prec*: glaucoma, prostatic hypertrophy, pregnancy B; *Adverse Rxs*: drowsiness*, dizziness*, dry mouth*, weakness, taste changes, fatigue, paresthesias, nausea, insomnia, blurred vision, seizures, hepatitis, tachycardia. Extended release formulation (Amrix, Cephalon) is available in 15 and 30 mg capsules and can be prescribed qd.

dantrolene (Dantrium, Proctor&Gamble) - [caps 25, 50, 100 mg; injection] *Indic/Dosage*: spasticity: start 25 mg qd, increase by 25 mg q4-7d, to max of 400 mg/d divided bid-qid (considered the oral agent of choice in TBI due to peripheral action and less CNS side effects); off-label for malignant hyperthermia: 2 mg/kg IV push until symptoms subside or cumulative dose of 10 mg/kg reached; also off-label for heat stroke and cocaine overdose rigidity; *Action*: reduces excitation-contraction coupling via reduction of sarcoplasmic reticulum Ca release; *Contra*: active liver disease, lactation; *Warn/Prec*: risk of hepatic dysfunction higher in women or if >35 yo, cardiomyopathy or pulmonary disease present, pregnancy C; *Adverse Rxs*: weakness*, malaise*, sedation*, dizziness*, nausea*, diarrhea*, acne-like rash, pruritus, h/a, insomnia, photosensitivity, fatal/nonfatal hepatotoxicity (most commonly 3–12 mos after initiation of tx, most cases resolve with d/c), seizures; *Monitoring*: baseline/periodic LFTs.

diazepam (Valium, Roche) - [tabs 2, 5, 10 mg; oral soln 5 mg/5 ml, 5 mg/1 ml; injection] *Indic/Dosage*: skeletal muscle spasticity due to local reflex spasm, UMN spasticity, athetosis, stiff-man syndrome: 2–10 mg po/IM tid-qid (geriatric pt 1–2.5 mg qd-bid); anxiety dosing similar to spasticity; EtOH withdrawal: initially 2–5 mg IV, repeat q3–4 hr prn; status epilepticus: 0.2–0.5 mg/kg/dose IV q15–30 min to a max of 30 mg; *Action*: proposed mechanism for antispasticity effect is a post-synaptic facilitation of spinal cord GABA w/o a direct GABA-mimetic effect; *Contra*: CNS depression, acute angle glaucoma; *Warn/Prec*: impaired liver/renal fxn, depression may worsen with use, psychotic reactions observed rarely, pregnancy D; *Adverse Rxs*: sedation*, "hangover"*, dizziness*, ataxia*, diplopia, hypotension, confusion, constipation, urinary retention/incontinence, anterograde amnesia, dependency, withdrawal syndrome, bone marrow suppression, rash, fever, hepatotoxicity, blood dyscrasias, injection site reaction (local pain and thrombophlebitis); apnea/cardiac arrest (rare, and typically only after IV administration or in elderly or medically ill pts).

metaxalone (Skelaxin, King Pharma) - [tab 400 mg, 800 mg] *Indic/Dosage*: relief of discomfort associated with acute, painful musculoskeletal conditions: 800 mg tid-qid; *Action*: not established, but may be due to general CNS depression; no direct action on contractile mechanism of striated muscle, motor end plate or nerve fiber; *Contra*: h/o anemias, significantly impaired renal/hepatic fxn; *Warn/Prec*: liver impairment, pregnancy (unknown); *Adverse Rxs:* drowsiness, paradoxic CNS excitation, nervousness, N/V, irritability, dizziness, rash, leukopenia, hemolytic anemia, jaundice.

methocarmabol (Robaxin, Schwarz Pharma) - [tab 500 mg, 750 mg; injection] *Indic/Dosage*: acute musculoskeletal pain, start 1500 mg po qid × 48–72 hrs, then 1000 mg po qid or 1500 mg po tid for maintenance; avail as IV or IM; FDA approved for spasm from tetanus; *Action*: unknown but skeletal muscle relaxant property presumed to be secondary to general CNS depression; *Warn/Prec*: caution in patients with renal or hepatic impairment; pregnancy C; avoid coadministration with alcohol or other CNS depressants; avoid coadministration with anticholinesterase; *Adverse Rxs*: somnolence*, dizziness*, abnormal taste, amnesia, blurred vision, confusion, diplopia, hypotension, fever, flushing, headache, hives, indigestion, insomnia, pruritus, nasal congestion, conjuctival injection, ataxia, seizures, bradycardia, vertigo, vomiting, jaundice, may darken urine.

tizanidine (Zanaflex, Acorda) - [tab 4 mg] *Indic/Dosage*: spasticity: no set dosing; sample regimen: start 2 mg qhs, then q3d increase to: 2 mg qam/2 mg qhs, then 2 mg qam/4 mg qhs etc till 4 mg tid; maximum dose is 36 mg/d; *Action*: central α-2 adrenergic agonist which reduces spasticity by increasing presynaptic inhibition of motoneurons; reportedly ~10% of the BP effects of clonidine; peak effects at 1–2 hrs after administration; *Warn/Prec*: impaired renal/hepatic fxn, pregnancy C; *Adverse Rxs*: somnolence*, weakness*, hypotension, dry mouth, dizziness, hepatotoxicity, severe bradycardia, hallucinations, asthenia, UTI, constipation, urinary frequency, flu-like symptoms, pharyngitis, rhinitis, increased spasms.

Neuropathic Pain

capsaicin (Zostrix, Medicis) - [cream 0.025%, 0.075%, both OTC] *Indic/ Dosage*: FDA approved for postherpetic neuralgia; commonly used for OA and neuropathic pain: apply a thin film to affected areas tid to qid; may require ongoing use for effect; experimental intravesical instillation inhibits contractions in neurogenic bladders; *Action*: evidence suggests capsaicin depletes the pain neurotransmitter substance P from unmyelinated peripheral neurons; *Warn/ Prec*: wash hands after application, avoid contact with eyes, avoid heating pads in treated areas; *Adverse Rxs*: local burning sensation*, which typically improves with repeated use, but may not be tolerated by some. Capsaicin 8% patch (Qutenza, NeurogesX) is approved for application by a physician for postherpetic neuralgia. Topical anesthetic is used before application of Qutenza, which is left on the skin for 60 minutes, after which cleaning gel and dry wipe are used after removal of the patch. Erythema, application site pain, pruritus, papules, inhalation of airborne capsaicin resulting in coughing and sneezing, and transient increase in blood pressure are potential side effects. Avoid use near eyes or mucous membranes.

carbamazepine (Tegretol, Novartis) - [tabs 100, 200 mg, XR (bid) tabs 100, 200, 300, 400 mg; oral susp 100 mg/5 ml] *Indic/Dosage*: epilepsy: start at 200 mg bid; trigeminal neuralgia: start 100 mg qd; off-label for neuropathic pain: start at 100 mg bid; max dose for all indications is 1200 mg/d, usually divided in tid doses, increase doses each wk by 200 mg/d; *Action*: unknown, but related to the TCAs; may be a result of Na channel blockade in rapidly firing neurons and reduced excitatory synaptic transmission in the trigeminal nucleus; *Contra*: TCA hypersensitivity, h/o bone marrow depression, concomitant use of MAOIs (or w/ in 14d of d/c); *Warn/Prec*: impaired liver/renal fxn, hyponatremia, pregnancy C, numerous drug interactions, Test for HLA-B*1502 allele prior to starting therapy in those with Chinese ancestry given 10-fold increased risk for toxic epidermal necrolysis and Stevens-Johnson syndrome; *Adverse Rxs*: (initially: dizziness*, ataxia*, drowsiness*, N/V*, but usually subside spontaneously w/in a wk), bone marrow suppression, hepato/nephrotoxicity, nystagmus, rash, Stevens-Johnson syndrome, arrhythmias; *Monitoring*: pre-tx CBC, BUN, LFTs, Fe, with periodic f/u (frequency guidelines not established).

gabapentin (Neurontin, Pfizer) - [caps 100, 300, 400 mg; tabs 600, 800 mg; soln 50 mg/ml] *Indic/Dosage*: partial seizures with or w/o secondary generalization: 300 mg qhs on day#1, titrate up by 100–300 mg q daily to q2d, continue to titrate as tolerated to effect, up to 1800 mg/d, although doses up to 3600 mg/d have reportedly been well-tolerated by some patients; off-label for neuropathic pain: titrate dose up by 300 mg every 2–3 days to effect; off-label second line tx for spasticity; *Action*: binds to the α2δ subunit of the voltage-gated calcium channel in the CNS, blocking channel action and thus calcium influx. Whether it is this mechanism that modulates pain is not entirely clear; *Warn/Prec*: impaired renal fxn, pregnancy C, d/c gradually over 1wk, (no known drug interactions); *Adverse Rxs*: (initially: somnolence*, dizziness*, ataxia*, but these usually resolve w/in 2wks of starting drug), fatigue*, nystagmus*, tremor, diplopia, nausea, nervousness, dysarthria, weight gain, leukopenia, thrombocytopenia, dyspepsia, depression, periorbital edema, myalgias.

lidocaine patch (Lidoderm, Endo) - [patch 5% (10 × 14 cm)] *Indic/Dosage*: FDA approved in 1999 to tx postherpetic neuralgia: apply up to 3 patches on intact skin over the most symptomatic area qd (12hrs on/12hrs off); off-label for other types of neuropathic pain; *Action*: diffusion of lidocaine into the local epidermis/dermis is thought to block conduction of impulses (inhibits Ca-mediated Na and K ion fluxes) and stabilize neuronal membranes; provides direct local analgesia w/o complete anesthetic block; *Warn/Prec*: do not reuse patches; avoid showers/swimming with patch on; when used appropriately, mean peak serum levels due to systemic absorption may reach about one-tenth the therapeutic level used for antiarrhythmia (these patches are safe); caution in pts with hepatic failure, or on anti-arrhythmics; pregnancy B; *Adverse Rxs*: initially: local erythema, edema, and or parasthesias, usually mild and resolve w/in minutes to 1 hr.

pregabalin (Lyrica, Pfizer) - [caps 25, 50, 75, 100, 150, 200, 225, 300 mg] *Indic/Dosage*: FDA approved for partial seizures, diabetic neuropathy, fibromyalgia and postherpetic neuralgia; *Action*: binds to the α2δ subunit of the voltage-gated calcium channel in the CNS, blocking channel action and thus calcium influx; primary difference between pregabalin and gabapentin is that while gabapentin's bioavailability declines with increased dosage, pregabalin's bioavailability remains linear; *Warn/Prec*: impaired renal fxn, pregnancy C, d/c gradually over 1wk, (no known drug interactions); Schedule V in the U.S.; *Adverse Rxs*: (initially: somnolence*, dizziness*, but these usually resolve w/in 2wks of starting drug), increased appetite*, nystagmus*.

topiramate (Topamax, Ortho-McNeil) - [tabs 25, 100, 200 mg, cap 15, 25 mg] *Indic/Dosage*: FDA approved in 1997 as an adjunct tx for partial onset seizures and mood stabilizer: start at 25 mg bid and increase daily dose 50 mg/wk until therapeutic (typically 200–400 mg/day); off-label use for neuropathic pain: no established dosing regimen, may start at 25 mg qhs with weekly increases of 25 mg/day; *Action*: Na channel blocker, but analgesic mechanisms unclear; *Warn/Prec*: pregnancy C; *Adverse Rxs*: somnolence*, dizziness*, vision problems (including acute angle glaucoma), unsteadiness*, changes in taste*, nausea, parasthesias, psychomotor slowing, nervousness, speech/memory problems, tremor, confusion.

Anti-Inflammatory

celecoxib (Celebrex, Pfizer) - [caps 100, 200 mg] *Indic/Dosage*: OA: 200 mg QD or 100 mg bid; RA: 100–200 mg bid; acute pain/ dysmenorrhea: 400 mg initially, followed by 200 mg if needed on first day, then 200 mg bid prn; *Action*: COX-2 selective NSAID; *Contra*: hyper-sensitivity to sulfonamides, ASA, NSAIDs; *Warn/Prec*: HTN, CHF, h/o GI bleed, renal insufficiency, monitor INRs closely with concomitant warfarin tx, pregnancy C, nasal polyps; *Adverse Rxs*: edema, GI distress/bleed, thrombocytopenia, nephro/hepatotoxicity, bronchospasm, agranulocytosis. Note: In the CLASS study (Silverstein FE: Celecoxib Long-term Arthritis Safety Study. JAMA 2000;284(10):1247–55), the annual incidence of upper GI ulcer complications (bleeding, perforation, obstruction) for celecoxib 200 bid vs. NSAIDs (ibuprofen 800 mg tid or diclofenac 75 mg bid) was 0.76% vs 1.45%; when combined with symptomatic ulcers, annual incidence was 2.08% vs 3.54% (p = 0.02).

diclofenac epolamine patch (Flector, Alpharma) – [topical patch, 1.3%, 10 cm × 14 cm] *Indic/Dosage*: acute pain due to minor strains, sprains, and contusions; 1 patch bid. *Action*: exact mechanism of action unknown; inhibits cyclooxygenase and lipoxygenase and reduces prostaglandin synthesis; *Contra*: treatment of peri-operative pain in the setting of coronary artery bypass graft (CABG) surgery, pregnancy 3rd trimester; *Adverse Rxs*: pruritus, dermatitis, headache, nausea, somnolence, cardiovascular thrombotic events, and GI adverse events including bleeding, ulceration, and perforation; *Warn/Prec*: should not be applied to damaged or non-intact skin and should not be worn when bathing or showering.

prednisone - [tabs 1, 2.5, 5, 10, 20, 50 mg; oral soln 5 mg/5 ml] *Indic/Dosage*: inflammatory disorders: 5–60 mg qd; Action: adrenocorticosteroid with glucocorticoid and mineralocorticoid activity; *Contra*: systemic fungal infection; *Warn/Prec*: seizure disorder, osteoporosis, CHF, DM, HTN, TB, impaired liver fxn, pregnancy C; *Adverse Rxs*: edema, mood swings, psychosis, adrenal insufficiency, immunosuppression, peptic ulcer, CHF, anaphylaxis, insomnia, anxiety, hypokalemia, osteoporosis, appetite change, h/a, dizziness, HTN, hyperglycemia, acne, cushingoid features, skin atrophy, ecchymosis, impaired wound healing, menstrual irregularities.

Miscellaneous

tramadol (Ultram, Johnson & Ortho-McNeil-Janssen) - [tab 50 mg] *Indic/Dosage*: FDA approved for moderate to moderately severe pain: 50–100 mg q4–6 hrs, not to exceed 400 mg/day (elderly: 300 mg/day; creatinine clearance <30 ml/min: dose q12hrs, 200 mg/day; hepatic impairment: 50 mg q12hrs); one 50 mg tab is roughly equivalent to one Tylenol #3; extended formulation may be taken qd-bid; *Action*: centrally acting synthetic non-opioid analogue of codeine that produces analgesia by weak μ-receptor agonism (has 10% of the affinity of codeine), serotonin/NE reuptake blockade, and enhancement of neuronal serotonin release; opioid-like CNS side-effects; *Contra*: acute EtOH intox; use with opioids, psychotropics or central analgesics; *Warn/Prec*: seizure disorder, head trauma, increased ICP, concomitant MAOI or SSRI, pregnancy C, acute abdominal conditions, opioid dependence; *Adverse Rxs*: vertigo*, nausea*, constipation, h/a, somnolence, vomiting, pruritus, asthenia, sweating, dry mouth, dyspepsia, diarrhea, syncope, orthostatic hypotension, tachycardia. Also available in long-acting formulation (Ultram ER, 100, 200, and 300 mg tab), may be taken q daily.

calcitonin nasal spray (Miacalcin, Novartis) - [metered dose intranasal spray 200 IU/activation (0.09 ml/puff)] *Indic/Dosage*: Used for osteoporosis in women who are at least 5 years after menopause. *Action*: potent inhibitor of osteoclastic bone resorption, and also has inherent analgesic properties which may make it useful in the early post fracture period; *Contra*: history of calcitonin allergy. nasal irritations. Safety in children, in pregnancy, or by nursing mothers not studied. *Adverse Rxs*:uncommon and are usually mild, but include flushing, rash, runny nose, nosebleed, bone pain and headaches, stomach upset.

Other Psychoactive Medications

modafinil (Provigil, Cepahalon) - [tabs 100, 200 mg] *Indic/Dosage*: improve wakefulness in patients with excessive sleepiness associated with narcolepsy, obstructive sleep apnea/hypopnea syndrome, and shift work sleep disorder; *Action*: unknown, but has wake-promoting actions like sympathomimetic agents including amphetamine and methylphenidate, although the pharmacologic profile is not identical to that of sympathomimetic amines; *Contra*: known hypersensitivity to modafinil; *Warn/Prec*: should be used in patients only with complete evaluation of sleepiness; may affect judgement, thinking, motor skills, impaired hepatic function; *Adverse Rxs*: headache*, nausea*, nervousness, rhinitis, diarrhea, back pain, anxiety, insomnia, dizziness, and dyspepsia.

valproic acid (Depakote, Abbott) - [cap 250 mg; oral soln 250 mg/5 ml; injection] *Indic/Dosage*: epilepsy or mania start 15 mg/kg qd, increase by 5–10 mg/d qwk to max of 60 mg/kg/d; migraines; reduce dose in elderly, do not d/c abruptly; off-label for neuropathic pain; *Action*: may be related to increased brain levels of GABA; *Contra*: hepatic dysfunction; *Warn/Prec*: impaired renal fxn, organic brain disease, hypoalbuminemia, pregnancy D; *Adverse Rxs*: GI distress*, anorexia, flu-like symptoms, somnolence, dizziness, ataxia, asthenia, tremor, diplopia, thrombocytopenia, bone marrow suppression, h/a, infection, menstrual irregularities, hair loss, wt changes, fatal hepatic failure (mostly infants), severe pancreatitis.

zonisamide (Zonegran, Eisai, Inc) - [caps 25, 100 mg] *Indic/Dosage*: off-label for certain forms of neuropathic pain but not approved for chidren under 16 years old; usual dose 100 mg qd, can gradually titrate up to 500 mg qd; *Action*: unknown, but possibly facilitates both dopaminergic and serotonergic neurotransmission, GABA receptor agonist; *Warn/Prec*: avoid in patients allergic to sulfa drugs, avoid driving or operating dangerous machinery, pregnancy category C, discontinue if rash develops, taper off slowly as abrupt discontinuation of Zonegran can cause seizures can cause metabolic acidosis; check sodium bicarbonate level prior to starting treatment and periodically after; *Adverse Rxs*: (usually in the first 4 weeks of therapy: anorexia*, somnolence*, dizziness*, headache*, nausea*, agitation*, irritability*), also: bloody or dark urine, coordination problems, decreased sweating or a rise in body temperature, depression, abdominal pain, fever, mouth sores, rash, sore throat, speech or language problems, kidney stones, tendency to bruise easily, unusual thoughts.

Migraine Medications

sumatriptan (Imitrex, GlaxoSmithKline) - [tabs 25, 50, 100 mg; nasal spray; injectable] *Indic/Dosage*: FDA approved, first generation triptan for migraine with or without aura (oral/nasal/injectable forms); will only treat headaches that have already begun, not for prevention or reduction of headache frequency or for use in management of hemiplegic or basilar migraine; injectable form for cluster headache attacks. Tabs: one 25, 50 or 100 mg tab (100 mg is the max single dose, with a max 24-hr dose of 200 mg; 100 mg tabs taken at least 2 hrs apart); with liver dz, max single dose is 50 mg. Nasal spray: usually 5 to 20 mg as soon as the attack begins, repeated only once, if needed, 2 hrs later; max single dose is 20 mg, max daily dose is 40 mg. Injection: max single dose is 6 mg injected under the skin; max 24-hr dose is two 6 mg injections, taken at least 1 hr apart; *Action*: 5-HT1D receptor agonist, causing cranial vessel constriction, inhibition of neuropeptide release and reduced transmission in trigeminal pain pathways; *Warn/Precs*: do not take >200 mg orally or >40 mg nasal spray in 24 hrs; must wait 2 hrs before second administration for either oral or nasal; do not take if MAOI use within the past 14 days or if ergot or triptan meds taken within the past 24 hrs; serotonin syndrome with concurrent MAOIs, SSRIs, TCAs or lithium; avoid in h/o seizure, CAD (MI, CVA, etc.) or risk factors of CAD (DM, menopause, smoking, obesity, high BP, high cholesterol), liver dz, ischemic bowel dz, or a headache that is different from other headache. Pregnancy C; *Adverse Rxs*: (adverse reactions are similar for all the triptans) parasthesiae*, neck pain/pressure*, feeling of heaviness*, malaise/fatigue*, vertigo*, warm/cold sensations*, nausea, vomiting, burning sensation, feeling of tightness, flushing, mouth and tongue discomfort, muscle weakness, numbness, redness at the site of injection, sinus or nasal discomfort (nasal spray), sore throat, unusual taste (nasal spray), wheezing. Treximet is a combination of 85 mg of sumitriptan and 500 mg of naproxen.

rizatriptan (Maxalt, Merck) - [regular/orally disintegrating tabs 5, 10 mg] *Indic/ Dosage*: second generation triptan for acute treatment of migraine attacks with or without aura; not intended for the prophylactic therapy of migraine or reduction of frequency or for use in the management of hemiplegic or basilar migraine; not yet approved for cluster headache. In comparison to first generation triptans, the second generation triptans have a higher oral bioavailability and longer plasma half-life. Usual dose is one 5 or 10 mg tab, followed by more taken at least 2 hrs apart (30 mg max daily dose); in patients receiving propranolol, the 5-mg dose should be used, up to a maximum of 3 doses in any 24-hour period; *Action*: selective 5-HT1B/1D receptor agonist; *Warn/Prec*: (similar to first generation triptans) ischemic heart disease, coronary artery vasospasm, hypertension, hypercholesterol; phenylketonuria; *Adverse Rxs*: (adverse reactions are similar for all the triptans) asthenia/fatigue*, somnolence*, pain/pressure sensations*, dizziness*, warm/cold sensations*, diarrhea*, vomiting*, decreased mental acuity*, euphoria*, tremor*, flushing*, blurred vision, anorexia, insomnia.

zolmitriptan (Zomig, AstraZeneca) - [tabs 2.5, 5 mg; orally disintegrating tabs 2.5, 5 mg; (2.5 mg tabs come in 6-tab packs; 5 mg tabs come in 3-tab packs); 5 mg single dose nasal spray, boxes of 6] *Indic/Dosage*: second generation triptan for acute treatment of migraine attacks with or without aura; not intended for the prophylactic therapy of migraine or reduction of frequency or for use in the management of hemiplegic or basilar migraine; not yet approved for cluster headache. In comparison to first generation triptans, the second generation triptans have a higher oral bioavailability and longer plasma half-life. Zomig should not be taken more frequently than every 2 hrs, with a max daily dose of 10 mg; *Action*: selective 5-HT$_{1B/1D}$ receptor agonist; *Warn/Prec*: (similar to first generation triptans) ischemic heart disease, coronary artery vasospasm, hypertension, hypercholesterol; phenylketonuria; *Adverse Rxs*: (adverse reactions are similar for all the triptans) parasthesia*, neck pain*, dizziness*, somnolence*, warm/cold sensations*, chest pain, nausea, feelings of heaviness, dry mouth.

Ch.11: COMMON OPIOID MEDICATIONS

Opium, an extract of *Papever somniferum* (the poppy plant), contains many alkaloids, including morphine, codeine, and papaverine. Opioids are morphine-like substances that mediate their effects via agonism or antagonism of CNS μ, κ, and δ receptors. The μ receptor mediates analgesia (via the μ1 receptor subtype) and respiratory depression (via brainstem μ2 receptors). The κ receptor (named after the agonist ketocyclazocine) produces analgesia with less respiratory depression than the μ receptor. The δ receptor results in similar effects as the μ receptor.

Naturally-occurring and semisynthetic agonists

Morphine (schedule II), a naturally-occurring phenanthrene series μ agonist. Given orally, it is completely absorbed in the small intestine and metabolized in liver to two metabolites: morphine-3-glucoronide (M3G), which contributes to most of the side effects, and morphine-6-glucoronide (M6G), which is ~100X more potent than morphine. Peak plasma levels are reached at ~1 hr for regular oral morphine, and 2.5 hrs for slow-release preparations. Profound effects can be seen in patients unable to renally excrete the M6G metabolite. Hydromorphone has been reported as a minor metabolite of morphine, especially in those taking high doses of morphine (Cone, 2006).

Codeine (schedule II, III or V) is a naturally-occurring pro-drug of morphine. ~10% is metabolized to the active analgesic morphine by hepatic enzyme CYP2D6. The rest either remains free, conjugates to form codeine-6-glucuronide (~70%), or converts to norcodeine (~10%). Hydrocodone has been reported as a minor metabolite of codeine, especially in those taking high doses of codeine (Oyler, 2000).

Diacetylmorphine (schedule I), or **heroin**, is a semisynthetic morphine derivative that is metabolized to morphine on first pass metabolism in the liver.

Hydromorphone (Dilaudid; schedule II) is a semisynthetic (hydrogenated ketone of morphine) μ agonist that is well absorbed orally or rectally, or can be delivered parenterally. It is lipid soluble, has less active metabolites and is sometimes recommended for patients with renal failure.

Hydrocodone compounds (Vicodin, Lortab, Norco, etc; schedule III) are weak μ agonists metabolized by CYP2D6 to the active metabolite hydromorphone. To deter excess use, hydrocodones are only available in combination with acetaminophen, aspirin, or NSAIDs, in USA.

Oxymorphone (Numorphan, Opana; schedule II) is a semisynthetic opioid derived from thebaine, previously only available parenterally. Immediate (Opana 5, 10 mg) and extended release (Opana ER: 5, 7.5, 10, 15, 20, 30, 40 mg) oxymorphone oral tablets were FDA-approved in 2006. Pregnancy Category C.

Oxycodone (schedule II) is a semisynthetic methylether of oxymorphone with μ agonist properties. Its oral bioavailability is ~60–87% of the parenteral dose. Oxycodone is essentially a prodrug that is extensively metabolized to inactive noroxycodone (via CYP3A4) and active oxymorphone (via CYP2D6).

Synthetic agonists

Fentanyl (Duragesic; schedule II) is 75–100X as potent as morphine, has high lipid solubility (penetrates the blood-brain barrier), and is hepatically metabolized by CYP3A4 to inactive metabolites norfentanyl as well as hydroxylated inactive metabolites hydroxyfentanyl and hydroxynorfentanyl. 2–48 hrs are required before drug delivered by transdermal patch is detected in blood. Fever (≥40° C) may increase absorption by a third. At therapeutic doses it offers less constipation, nausea, and sedation than morphine.

An oral transmucosal (berry-flavored) "lollipop" version of fentanyl (Actiq) as well as buccal tablet (Fentora) are available for breakthrough cancer pain who are already receiving and tolerant (≥60 mg morphine/day or equianalgesic equivalent for ≥1 wk) to opioid therapy.

Sufentanil is a thienyl derivative of fentanyl that has a 30X greater affinity for opioid receptors and is 5–10X more potent than fentanyl. *Alfentanil* is a ultra-short acting congener of fentanyl that is one-tenth as potent, but has a more rapid analgesic effect and a shorter elimination t½ than fentanyl. It is metabolized by CYP3A3/4. Erythromycin can decrease clearance by 50%. It is indicated for incremental injections, continuous infusion, or anesthesia induction. *Remifentanil* is the shortest-acting opioid clinically available, with pharmacokinetics unaltered in renal or liver disease, but possibly with age. It is prepared with glycine and is not for intrathecal/epidural use, due to risk of motor impairment.

Meperidine (Demerol; schedule II) is a fast-acting phenylpiperidine that metabolizes to normeperidine (renally cleared), which has half the analgesic properties of meperidine, but lowers the seizure threshold. Notably, naloxone does not reverse the seizure, but may in fact precipitate seizure. Meperidine's purportedly decreased spasmodic effect on the sphincter of Oddi relative to morphine is debatable. During labor, meperidine increases contractions, and there is less respiratory depression of the newborn than with morphine. Use should not exceed 600 mg/24 hrs (assuming normal renal function). Avoid in hemodialysis patients.

Methadone (Dolophine; schedule II) is a phenylheptylamine that is less sedating and euphoric yet more potent than morphine. Plasma protein binding results in a long, albeit unpredictable, t½ (13–100 hrs). It is metabolized by CYP3A4. If dosed more frequently than the t½, the drug accumulates. A steady state is usually achieved in 2–3 days (vs. hrs for morphine). It is also a weak noncompetitive NMDA-receptor agonist, which may potentially be responsible for regulating drug dependence and tolerance.

Levorphanol (Levo-dromoran; schedule II) is a morphonan with affinity to μ, κ, and δ opioid receptors. It is considered a full κ agonist. The L-isomer is analgesic; O-methyl derivative of the D-isomer (dextromethorphan) is an antitussive. The duration of analgesia lasts 4–6 hrs, but t½ is 12–16 hrs and repeat dosing can lead to drug accumulation. It is a weak noncompetitive NMDA receptor antagonist but is considered a more potent NMDA antagonist than racemic methadone.

Propoxyphene (Darvon, Darvocet; schedule IV) is a weak μ agonist; only the d-isomer of the racemic mixture is analgesic. It is hepatically metabolized by CYP2D6 to the active norpropoxyphene (t½, 30 hrs); hepatic dysfunction can result in toxicity. Propoxyphene can decrease carbamezepine metabolism. Side effects include depression of cardiac conduction, pulmonary edema, hallucinations, and delusions. In the United States, FDA has recommended against continued prescribing and use of propoxyphene because of concern for cardiac arrhythmia.

Tapentadol (Nucynta, Schedule II) is a centrally-acting synthetic analgesic with μ-agonist activity and norepinephrine reuptake inhibition. Typical dose 50, 75 or 100 mg po q4-6 hrs. Max dose 600 mg/d. Caution in patients at risk for raised CSF pressure, seizure disorder, hepatic and renal impairment. Potential for serotonin syndrome. Majority of tapentadol metabolism is via conjugation with glucuronic acid to produce glucuronides. No significant inhibition or induction of CYP450 enzymes. Contraindicated in those with impaired pulmonary function, paralytic ileus or concomitant use of MAOI within 14 days. Pregnancy Category C. Not recommended for nursing mothers. Available in 50, 75, 100 mg tabs.

Partial agonists and agonist-antagonists offer less efficacious analgesia, but also less respiratory depression and (theoretically) less abuse than pure μ agonists.

Buprenorphine (Temgesic, Buprenex, Subutex; schedule III) is a highly lipophilic semisynthetic thebaine-derivative partial μ agonist. When given IM, it is 30X more potent than morphine, with the analgesic effect occurring in 45–60 mins (duration 3–14 hrs). Euphoria is less, but sedation is greater than with morphine. The dose-response curve is bell-shaped: with increasing doses, κ antagonism increases and analgesia is reduced, but side effects, such as respiratory depression, also have a ceiling effect. The sublingual form is long-acting (can be dosed every other day) and is often used in the management of opioid dependence. Subutex and Suboxone (formulation that combines naloxone with buprenorphine) can be prescribed for treatment of opioid addiction in USA if the treating provider has obtained a special federal waiver.

Pentazocine (Talwin; schedule IV), a derivative of benzomorphinan, is a weak competitive μ antagonist and κ agonist. Adverse effects include hallucinations and confusion. In patients on morphine, pentazocine does not reverse respiratory depression, but can cause withdrawal. Naloxone has been combined with pentazocine to curb abuse (pentazocine + tripelennamine, an antihistamine, can result in euphoria).

Butorphanol (Stadol; schedule IV), or 14-hydroxymorphinan, is a κ agonist and μ antagonist. Extensive first-pass metabolism requires IV, IM, or intranasal routes. Analgesia is superior to pentazocine and equivalent to morphine, while side effects are less (a 2 mg ceiling on respiratory depression).

Nalbuphine (Nubain; schedule IV), derived from oxymorphone and naloxone, acts via κ agonism and μ antagonism.

Opioid drug interactions
- Alcohol or CNS depressants – increased CNS and respiratory depression, hypotension
- Anticholinergics – severe constipation/ paralytic ileus
- Antidiarrheals – severe constipation / CNS depression
- Antihypertensives – hypotensive effects potentiated
- Buprenorphine – precipitate withdrawal in dependent patients
- Carbamazepine – concurrent use w/ propoxyphene can decrease metabolism of carbamazepine, resulting in toxic serum levels
- Hydroxyzine – increased CNS and respiratory depression, increased analgesia
- Metoclopramide – opioids antagonize metoclopromide GI motility effects
- MAO-inhibitors – especially with meperidine, can be fatal (coma, HTN, seizure, death)
- Naloxone – antagonizes the analgesic, CNS and respiratory depressive effects of opioids
- Naltrexone – antagonizes opioid effects
- Neuromuscular blocking agents – increased respiratory depression
- Tobacco smoking – increases metabolism of propoxyphene leading to decreased therapeutic effect
- Chronic Phenytoin or Rifampin – increase methadone metabolism, may cause withdrawal
- Zidovudine – morphine may reduce clearance, causing toxicity

Side effects of opioids include constipation, sedation, respiratory depression, pruritus, nausea, and urinary retention. Opioids can also result in endocrine effects including: central hypogonadism; decreased hypothalamic GNRH, pituitary LH, and possibly FSH; decreased testicular testosterone and ovarian estradiol; decreased testicular interstitial fluid; loss of libido; depression, anxiety, fatigue; loss of muscle mass and strength; amenorrhea, irregular menses, galactorrhea; osteoporosis and fractures; cortisol deficiency; and growth hormone deficiency.

Ref: **Cone EJ, et al.** Evidence of morphine metabolism to hydromorphone in pain patients chronically treated with morphine. *J Anal Tox* 2006;30:1; **Oyler JM, et al.** Identification of hydrocodone in human urine following controlled codeine administration. *J Anal Tox* 2000;24:530; **Miyoshi HR, et al.** Systemic Opioid Analgesics, Chapter 84. In: Loeser, et al., eds. Bonica's Management of Pain, 3rd ed. Philadelphia, LWW, 2001; **Inturrisi CE, et al.** Narcotic analgesics in the management of pain. In: Kuhar M, et al., eds. Analgesics: neurochemical, behavioral, and chemical perspectives. New York, Raven Press, 1994: 257–98; **Cherny NI.** Opioid analgesics: comparative features and prescribing guidelines. *Drugs* 1996;51:713; **Katz N, Mazer NA.** The impact of opioids on the endocrine system. *Clin J Pain* 2009;25:170; **Abs R, et al.** Endocrine consequences of long-term intrathecal administration of opioids. *J Clin Endo Metab* 2000;85:2215; **Drug Information for the Health Care Professional,** USP DI, 17th ed., Vol.I, 1997;2206–9.

Formulation of selected commonly used opioids

morphine (Roxanol, Oramorph SR, MSIR), available as po, IM, IV, PR. Generic/trade: tabs, immediate release: 15 & 30 mg. Trade: caps: 15 & 30 mg. Generic/trade: oral soln (Roxanol) 10 mg/5 mL, 10 mg/2.5 mL, 20 mg/5 mL, 20 mg/mL & 100 mg/5 mL. Rectal suppositories: 5, 10, 20 & 30 mg. Controlled release: MS Contin, Oramorph SR: 15, 30, 60 & 100 mg; 200 mg (MS Contin only). Controlled relase caps (Kadian): 10, 20, 30, 50, 60, 80, 100 & 200 mg. Extended release caps (Avinza): 30, 45, 60, 75, 90 & 120 mg.

codeine 0.5–1 mg/kg up to 15–60 mg PO/IM/IV/SC q4–6h. Avoid IV in children. Generic tabs 15, 30 & 60 mg. Oral soln 15 mg/5 mL, cleared by CYP2D6.

fentanyl patch (Duragesic), available in 12 μg/hr, 25 μg/hr, 50 μg/hr, 75 μg/hr, and 100 μg/hr patches.

hydromorphone (Dilaudid, Dilaudid-5) available as po, IM, SC, PR. Adults 2–4 mg po q4–6 h; 0.5–2 mg IM/SC or slow IV q4–6 h; 3 mg PR q6–8 h. Peds age 12 or under: 0.03–0.08 mg/kg po q4–6 h prn; 0.015 mg/kg/dose IV q4–6 h prn. Generic/trade: tabs 2, 4 & 8 mg (8 mg trade scored), liquid 5 mg/5 mL, suppositories 3 mg. Trade only: tabs 1 & 3 mg

hydrocodone (various formulations, available only with acetaminophen or NSAID in USA). More commonly used formulations include Vicodin (hydrocodone/acetaminophen 5 mg/500 mg), Vicodin ES (7.5/500), Vicodin HP (10/660), Lortab (avail as 2.5/500, 5/500, 7.5/500 or 10/500), Norco (10/325), Norco 5/325, Norco 7.5/325, Lorcet Plus (7.5/650), Lorcet 10/650. Also available as vicoprofen in combination with ibuprofen (hydrocodone 7.5 mg/ibuprofen 200 mg) and in elixir (Lortab elixir, hydrocodone 7.5 mg/acetaminophen 500 per 5 ml)

methadone (Dolophine 5 & 10 mg; liquid form available for treatment of heroin addiction)

oxycodone (various formulation, available alone or in combination with acetaminophen or NSAID). Percocet (oxycodone/acetaminophen 5 mg/325 mg) and Percodan (oxycodone/aspirin 5/325). Long acting formulation, Oxycontin, is available in 10, 15, 20, 30, 40, 60 & 80 mg tablets in USA.

Opioid equianalgesic table*

Drug	IM/IV (mg)	Oral (mg)	Dur (hr) IM / po	½-life (hr)**
Morphine	10	30	3–5 / 3–4	2.0–3.5
Codeine	120	180	4–6 / 3–4	3
Hydromorphone	1.5	7.5	3–4 / 4–6	2–3
Hydrocodone		30	/ 4–6	2–4
Oxycodone		20	/ 4–6	3–4.5
Oxymorphone	1	10	3–6 / 4–6	6–10
Levorphanol	2	4	3–6 / 3–6	12–16
Meperidine	75	300	2–3 / 2–3	2–4
Fentanyl	0.1		0.75–1.0	1.7 min

Peak for most opioids: 0.5–1 hr via IM, 1–2 hr via po. *When switching opioids, take into account incomplete cross-tolerance and reduce the dose of the new drug by 25–50%.
**Assuming normal hepatorenal function.

Conversion from an opioid to methadone in the treatment of chronic pain depends on the morphine equivalent dosage, as shown below:

Morphine equivalent   Methadone conversion rate (chronic pain)

<100 mg	3:1 (i.e., 30 mg morphine = 10 mg methadone)
101–300 mg	5:1
301–600 mg	10:1
601–800 mg	12:1
801–1000 mg	15:1
>1000 mg	20:1

Morphine to Fentanyl transderm conversion***

oral morphine (mg/24h)	fentanyl (mcg/hr)
60–134	25
135–224	50
225–314	75
315–404	100
405–494	125
495–584	150
585–674	175
675–764	200
765–854	225
855–944	250
945–1034	275
1035–1124	300

***from Duragesic package insert. This table should not be used to convert from fentanyl patch to other therapies because this conversion to fentanyl patch is conservative. Using this table to other analgesic therapies can overestimate the dose of the new agent.

Ref: Pain Management Guide and Analgesic & Opioid Conversion Table. VA Greater Los Angeles Healthcare System, 2005.

Ch.12: PATIENT CONTROLLED ANESTHESIA (PCA)

Patient controlled analgesia (PCA) utilizes a programmable pump that allows patients to self-administer parenteral opioids on demand. Used in hospitals since 1971, PCA is an effective and well-tolerated means of managing acute pain, including post-operative pain, as well as cancer, burn, and sickle-cell crisis pain.

Compared to other administration routes (po/sc/IM), PCA can provide better overall pain relief, greater patient control over pain, rapid treatment of incident pain (for dressing changes, etc.), more predictable drug absorption, lower drug consumption, and decreased nursing staff workload. Moreover, differences between patients in drug metabolism and effectiveness are minimized since each patient manages their PCA to the desired effect.

Conditions favorable for PCA use include the need for rapid opioid titration; moderate-severe pain; and frequent changes in pain intensity (e.g., incident pain). PCA therapy should be expected to be required for >48 hrs. ***Contraindications/relative contraindications for PCA*** include decreased comprehension/understanding (e.g., dementia, delirium, language barriers, age <7 years), poor or limited hand function, significant sleep apnea, severe lung disease, and poor renal function.

PCA variables and terminology

Choice of drug and administration route (IV, epidural, or subcutaneous); commonly used drugs with typical doses include:

Drug (concentration)	Bolus dose	Lockout interval
Morphine* (1mg/ml)	0.5–4.0 mg	6–15 mins
Hydromorphone (0.2 mg/ml)	0.1–0.6 mg	6–15 mins
Fentanyl (10 mg/ml)	0.02–0.10 mg	6–15 mins
Meperidine* (10 mg/ml)	5.0–25.0 mg	6–15 mins

*In renal failure, morphine and meperidine byproducts may accumulate.

- Loading dose - an initial bolus to make the patient comfortable.
- Infusion rate - continuous (basal) infusion that may be given with or without doses on demand. Basal infusions can aide sleep, improve pain control after very painful surgeries (e.g., GI, thoracic), and are often used in the setting of chronic opioid use. Disadvantages include the need for closer supervision and the loss of the intrinsic safety of PCA.
- Demand dose - the dose delivered by bolus when triggered by the patient. Triggering by proxy (e.g., nurse, family) increases the risk of adverse events and should be avoided.
- Lockout interval - is the amount of time a PCA pump is refractory to additional triggers after a bolus dose is delivered. It is commonly set at 6, 10, or 15 mins. Hourly and 4 hr maximal doses offer additional safeguards.

Managing inadequate pain relief with PCA

- Exclude medical or post-operative complications.
- Interrogate the PCA pump: if trigger attempts greatly exceed therapeutic boluses (e.g., by a factor of ≥3), discuss the pain with the patient. If VAS >5, increase the demand dose by 25%.
- Re-evaluate the patient in 2 hrs. If pain relief is still inaequate, increase the demand dose another 25%.

- Re-evaluate again in 2 hrs. If pain relief is suboptimal, derease lockout interval by 25%.

Common side effects and their treatments
- Nausea/vomiting, and constipation are treated per usual means.
- Pruritus - consider reducing basal rate or PCA bolus, and/or give diphenhydramine (Benadryl) 25–50 mg IV or po q 6 hrs PRN.
- Respiratory depression is treated with naloxone (0.4 mg ampule in 10 ml normal saline, given in 0.5 ml increments IV push q 2 mins), titrated to respiratory rate and wakefulness. Onset of action is 2–3 mins; the effects last up to 1 hr. Excessive naloxone can cause withdrawal, seizures, and severe pain.

Conversion from PCA to oral medications
- Should be performed ≥24 hrs before discharge. The patient should be tolerating clear liquids and performing ADLs with minimal assist. The pain should be rated ≤4 on VAS.
- Calculate total PCA opioid usage over 24 hrs and convert to an oral dose using an equianalgesic chart, adjusting for incomplete cross-tolerance (e.g., reducing dose by 25–50% if switching opioids). Wait ≥90 mins after giving short-acting orals (or for the peak effect for long acting orals, e.g., ~6 hrs for morphine) before discontinuing the PCA.

Refs: Kerri-Szanto M. Apparatus for demand analgesia. *Can Anaesth Soc J* 1971;18:581; **Smythe M.** PCA: a review. *Pharmacotherapy* 1992;12:132.

Ch.13: INJECTION AGENTS

Local anesthetics: Reversibly block sodium channels to impede nerve conduction. Generally, smaller unmyelinated fibers are more susceptible to local anesthetics than larger myelinated fibers. Nociceptors are blocked first, then proprioception/light touch, followed by motor fibers

Duration of action:
procaine - lasts about 30–90 mins.
lidocaine - lasts about 2–4 hrs.
mepivacaine - lasts about 3–5 hrs.
bupivicaine - lasts about 6–12 hrs.

Types:
Amino esters (structurally related to paraaminobenzoic acid, which is a known allergen; allergic reactions have occurred with the use of tetracaine). Examples: cocaine, procaine, chlorprocaine, tetracaine.

Amino amides (have two "i" in their generic name)
Examples: lidocaine, bupivacaine, mepivacaine, prilocaine, etidocaine, ropivacaine.

Steroids: Corticosteroids, such as dexamethasone and prednisone, act by binding to receptors which then act to modulate gene transcription in target tissues. Corticosteroids bind with receptors in numerous systems throughout the body, including the CNS (readily crossing the blood brain barrier), GI, musculoskeletal, and many other systems. Thus it is not surprising that corticosteroids are prone to producing side effects when administered at the doses to achieve specific desired effect(s). When given orally in doses that are effective for pain, they can result in acute side effects such as mood and behavioral changes, headaches, convulsions, insomnia, GI upset, acute steroid myopathy, neuropathy, hypertension, and hyperglycemia, etc. These side effects are the basis for giving steroids by injection (local delivery) instead of orally (systemic delivery). Injected steroids are believed to result in local analgesia, anti-inflammatory effects, neural tissue conduction suppression, and potentially disease-modifying effects. Steroids injected under fluoroscopic guidance (for maximal accuracy) are now cornerstone of interventional pain management. Common corticosteroids used for injections include, from least to most potent (relative potencies in parentheses): hydrocortisone (1), methylprednisolone (5), triamcinolone (5), betamethasone (25), and dexamethasone (25). The relative duration of action in intra-articular injections, from shortest to longest, is: hydrocortisone acetate (<1 wk), triamcinolone acetate, methylprednisolone acetate, betamethasone acetate, and triamcinolone hexacetonide (~3–6 wks). Suggested dosing guidelines are listed below:

joint	triamcinolone	methylprednisolone	betamethasone
knee	40 mg	40 mg	6 mg
shoulder	40 mg	40 mg	6 mg
bursa	10–20 mg	10–20 mg	1.5–3 mg
finger	5–10 mg	5–10 mg	1.5 mg
tendon sheath	5–10 mg	5–10 mg	1.5 mg

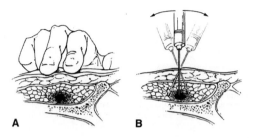

Figure 13   Trigger point injection.

Botulinum toxin (BTX): Botulinum toxin (BTX) - BTX inhibits the release of acetylcholine at the neuromuscular junction. BTX may also act on substance P and other factors (Wenzel, 2004), which may be an additional basis for its observed analgesic effects.

Trigger Point Injections: Indicated for relief of pain associated with myofascial pain syndrome. Frequently, a taut band of muscle spasm is palpated. Inject 1 to 2 ml of local anesthetic into and around the trigger point with a 25-gauge 1½ inch needle, aspirating prior to injection. Dry needling the surrounding area may also be performed in attempt to break up the taut muscle tissue spasm.

Ref: Simons DG, Travell JG, Simons L. Travell and Simons'. Myofascial Pain and Dysfunction:The Trigger Point Manual: The Lower Extremities. 2nd ed. Philadelphia, LWW, 1999. **Wenzel RG.** Pharmacology of Botulinim Toxin Serotype A. *Am J Health Sys Pharm.* 2004;61:S5. **Figure credits: 13.** Courtesy of **Loeser JD, et al.**, eds. *Bonica's Management of Pain,* 3rd ed. Philadelphia, LWW, 2001, with permission.

52

Ch.14: SELECTED PERIPHERAL INJECTIONS

Note: Becuase of the potential risks involved, injections should be performed only by those experienced with the procedure, or under direct supervision of those who have extensive experience with the procedure. More than one method to perform the injections may exist. The following are suggested injections as described in literature and various textbooks. The information contained herein is abridged; please refer to authoritative literature for more detailed information.

Supraorbital/trochlear nerve: *Indications:* migraine headaches and neuropathy. The terminal divisions of the ophthalmic branch of the trigeminal nerve are the supraorbital and supratrochlear nerve, which supply skin and conjunctiva sensation. *Technique:* perpendicular to the orbital rim above the eyebrow, the supraorbital foramen is palpated and then a needle is inserted toward the foramen without entering it so as to avoid nerve injury. 2–3 ml of local anesthetic is injected. Concerns include hematoma, supraorbital artery laceration.

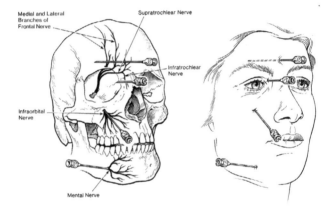

Medial and Lateral
Branches of
Frontal Nerve

Supratrochlear Nerve

Infratrochlear
Nerve

Infraorbital
Nerve

Mental Nerve

Figure 14a   Supraorbital/trochlear nerve block.

Maxillary nerve: *Indications:* trigeminal neuralgia, neuropathic pain, atypical facial pain. The maxillary nerve provides sensation to the face. It exits the foramen rotundum and traverses the superior pterygopalatine fossa. It enters the floor of the orbit at the inferior infraorbital fissure. *Technique:* palpate the mandibular notch and enter the pterygoid plate. The needle is redirected 45° to the eye until paresthesia is obtained. Concerns include CSF injection, orbital injection, hemorrhage, and hematoma.

Trigeminal nerve: *Indications:* trigeminal neuralgia. The trigeminal nerve is composed of the ophthalmic, maxillary and mandibular divisions, which provide sensation to the face, cornea, and motor control for mastication. *Technique:* inject the Gasserian ganglion at Meckel's cave; start 1 cm lateral to the mouth in the midpupillary line, with a 22-gauge 3.5 inch needle. Local anesthetic or neurolytic agent is injected in 1/4 ml increments until desired analgesic effect is achieved.

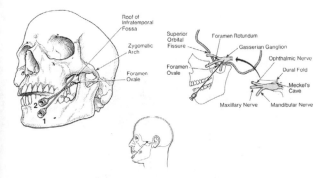

Figure 14b Trigeminal nerve block.

Concerns include technically challenging nature of the procedure, pain, possible CSF injection.

Glossopharyngeal nerve: *Indications:* Atypical face pain, neuralgia, pharyngeal cancer, refractory hiccups. It is the 9th cranial nerve with both sensory and motor components. It exits the jugular foramen between the internal carotid artery and inferior jugular vein. It provides sensation to the posterior 1/3rd of the tongue, tonsils, pharynx and auditory canal. *Technique:* There are two injection techniques using a 25-guage 2 inch needle. With the external technique, the needle is inserted at the midpoint of mastoid and the angle of the mandible. With the internal technique the needle is inserted at a right angle to the skin, at a depth of 2–3 cm until the styloid process is contacted and then walked off posteriorly. Concerns for injection include intravascular injection, which could result in seizures or dysphagia.

Occipital nerve: *Indications:* tension headaches, whiplash injuries, occipital neuralgia. It is a branch of the posterior ramus of the second cervical nerve and

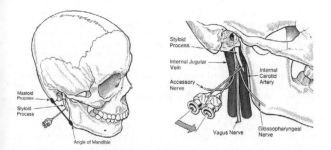

Figure 14c Glossopharyngeal nerve block.

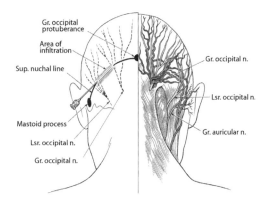

Figure 14d   Occipital nerve block.

supplies the posterior scalp. *Technique:* palpate the superior nuchal line, midway between the external occipital protuberance and the mastoid process. Locate the nerve by palpating the occipital artery and insert the needle just lateral. The needle is advanced to bone or paresthesia then retracted 1–2 mm. If negative for blood on aspiration, 2–3 ml of local anesthetic is injected along with steroid. Concerns include post-injection ecchymosis and hematoma as well as inadvertent placement of the needle into the foramen magnum and subarachnoid administration of local anesthetic.

Suprascapular nerve: *Indications:* shoulder pain secondary to OA, rotator cuff lesions, adhesive capsulitis or shoulder arthroscopy. *Technique:* 22-gauge 1½ inch needle is inserted 1–2 cm superior to the midpoint of the spine of the scapula towards the suprascapular notch until paresthesias are noted. 5–10 ml of anesthetic are injected. Concerns for injection include pneumothorax, infection, intravascular injection, seizure, muscle atrophy.

Brachial plexus: *Indications:* surgery of the shoulder or arm, shoulder dislocation or extremity level. The root level is at the intrascalenes, trunk level is supraclavicular, cord level is infraclavicular, branch level is at the axillary artery. *Technique:* at the interscalene groove at approximately C6 at the cricoid cartilage and posterior border of the sternocleidomastoid, a 25-gauge 1½ inch needle is advanced at a 45 degree angle until paresthesia to shoulder, arm occurs. Inject approximately 20 ml of local anesthetic. There are other techniques for brachial plexus injection including infraclavicular and axillary approaches. Concern is for possible vascular injection, thrombus, hematoma.

Intercostal nerve: *Indications:* rib fractures, chest wall metastases, post-thoracotomy pain. The intercostal nerves are the anterior rami of the first 11 thoracic spinal nerves. *Technique:* pt is placed in a semilateral position. Injection is performed at the posterior axillary line 5–7 cm lateral to the vertebral spinous process. A 25-gauge ½ inch needle, or longer if needed, is walked off to just below the rib and then advanced 2–3 mm forward. 3 ml of local anesthetic is then

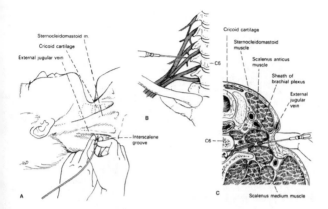

Figure 14e Brachial plexus block.

injected with epinephrine at each rib. Concerns include pneumothorax, intravascular injection, seizures, infection, bleeding.

Ulnar nerve: *Indications:* compression or entrapment neuropathies at the elbow or wrist. The ulnar nerve innervates intrinsic hand muscles, flexor carpi ulnaris and the ulnar portion of the flexor digitorum profundus. It also supplies sensory innervation to the ulnar aspect of the palm and the 4th and 5th digits. *Technique:* At the elbow, between the triceps and brachialis 5 cm above the medial epicondyle in line with the apex of the axilla, a 25-gauge 1½ inch needle is inserted perpendicularly to the humerus. An injection can also be performed at the ulnar groove with the needle inserted at the medial epicondyle, below and anterior to the olecranon tip. Injection at the wrist has less risk. The pisiform and flexor carpi ulnaris (FCU) tendon are palpated. From a volar approach a 25-gauge 1 inch needle is inserted to either side of the FCU 1 cm proximal to the pisiform. An ulnar approach can be used by inserting the needle at the medial wrist, directing it radially under the FCU. Injection at Guyon's canal can be done by palpating the pisiform and hook of the hamate and placing a needle between at the distal wrist crease, radial to the pisiform, angling it distally so it is ulnar to the hook of the hamate. Concerns include intravascular injection, nerve injury, paresthesias.

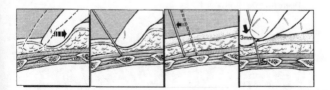

Figure 14f Intercostal nerve block.

56

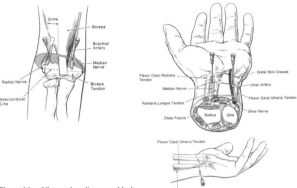

Figure 14g Ulnar and median nerve block.

Median nerve: *Indications:* entrapment neuropathies. The median nerve inner-vates the forearm flexor group, most of the thenar eminence and cutaneous dis-tribution of the lateral 3½ digits. *Technique:* median nerve block at the elbow is done with the elbow extended at the intersection of the biceps tendon and elbow crease, palpate the brachial artery and insert a 25-gauge 1½ inch needle medial to the artery. With a median nerve block at the pronator teres, the needle is placed 2–2.5 cm below the midpoint between the medial epicondyle and biceps tendon or at the point of maximal tenderness. A median nerve block at the wrist is done with the forearm supinated. A 27-gauge 5/8 inch needle is inserted proxi-mal to the distal wrist crease and medial to the flexor carpi radialis tendon at a 30° angle. Concerns include intravascular injection, nerve injury, paresthesias.

Radial nerve: *Indications:* distal radial neuropathies, entrapments. The radial nerve innervates the extensor forearm compartment and supplies sesnsation to posterior forearm and the dorsum of the hand. *Technique:* Radial nerve block at the elbow is performed at the elbow crease lateral to the biceps tendon and me-dial to the brachioradialis muscle. A 25-gauge 2 inch needle is inserted to bone at the lateral epicondyle and then withdrawn 1 cm. Concern of nerve injury.

Digital nerve block: *Indications:* minor procedures, compression neuropathies. The digital nerves originate from the median and ulnar nerves. *Technique:* a

Figure 14h Digital nerve block.

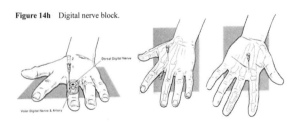

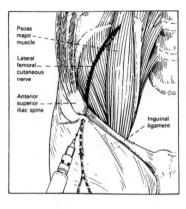

Figure 14i Lateral femoral cutaneous nerve block.

25-gauge 1 inch needle is inserted on the dorsolateral and dorsomedial aspect at the base of the finger and passed anteriorly beyond the base of the distal phalanx. Inject 1 ml while withdrawing to block the volar nerve and then inject 0.5 ml just beneath the point of entry for the dorsal nerve. Concerns include nerve injury, paresthesia.

Lateral femoral cutaneous nerve: *Indications:* meralgia paresthetica (burning pain, numbness and tingling in the anterolateral thigh). LFC nerve supplies sensation to the anterolateral thigh. It can become entrapped as it passes under the inguinal ligament. *Technique:* palpate the ASIS. Insert 25-gauge 1½ inch needle 2 cm medial and 2 cm caudal to ASIS. Proceed through the fascia until a pop is felt, then inject up to 10 ml of local anesthetic and steroid in a fanwise manner. Concerns include possible dysesthesia or hypoesthesia.

Ilioinguinal nerve block: *Indications:* posthernrhaphy pain caused by trauma to the genitofemoral nerve, diagnostic block, testicular pain. Supplies sensation to the medial thigh and groin. *Technique:* palpate the ASIS, insert a 22-gauge 1½ inch needle, create a skin wheal 2 cm medial to the ASIS, and infiltrate muscle layers toward the umbilicus with up to 5 ml of local anesthetic. Concerns include nerve injury, paresthesia.

Genitofemoral nerve block: *Indications:* groin or testicular pain unrelieved by ilioinguinal block. The nerve emerges on the anterior surface of the psoas. The genital branch enters the spermatic cord and supplies the cremaster; the femoral branch supplies a small area of the skin of the thigh. *Technique:* place patient supine and inject up to 5 ml of of local anesthetic around the spermatic cord at the base of the scrotum. Concerns include vascular injection, nerve damage.

Piriformis syndrome: *Indications:* entrapment pain with referred pain from the SI joint to the proximal 2/3 of the postero-lateral thigh. The piriformis muscle inserts into the anterior surface of the sacrum, exits the greater sciatic foramen and attaches at the greater trochanter. It is innervated by S1 and S2 and is a lateral hip rotator and abductor. *Technique:* locate the mid-point between the greater trochanter and the posterior superior iliac spine. Use 22-gauge

58

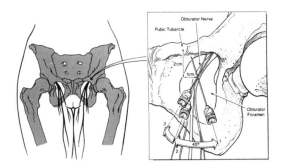

Figure 14j Obturator nerve block.

3½ inch spinal needle to enter the skin at 90 degree angle. Placement can be confirmed with contrast solution under fluoroscopy. Approximately 3 ml of local anesthetic and steroid are injected. Concerns include bleeding, hematoma, infection, sciatic nerve damage. Transvaginal approach is an alternative.

Greater Trochanteric Bursa: *Indications:* for acute or chronic bursitis follow-ing trauma or overuse. The bursa lies over the greater trochanter of the femur and is frequently tender to palpation. *Technique:* the pt lies on the unaffected side with the lower leg flexed and the upper leg extended. The tender point is identified. The greater trochanter is palpated and a 25-gauge 1½ inch needle is used to contact the os, then retracted 0.5 cm. Steroid and local anesthetic are injected after negative aspiration.

Obturator nerve: *Indications:* surgical procedures and adductor spasticity. Obturator nerve originates from the L2–L4 ventral nerve roots, exiting the ob-turator canal, supplying the adductor thigh muscles and sensation of the medial thigh. *Technique:* palpate the pubic tubercle and moving 2 cm lateral and 2 cm caudal, insert a 25-gauge 1½ inch needle until reaching os of the superior ramus. Walk off in an inferio-caudal direction into the obturator canal. Obturator nerve is located 2–3 cm past the initial contact with the pubic ramus. Inject up to 10 ml of local anesthetic. Concerns include arterial injection, hematoma, pelvic cavity injection.

Trigger finger injection: *Indications:* painful clicking and locking of fingers or thumb with inability to actively extend the joint, caused by nodule in the flexor tendon sheath. *Technique:* hand is placed on the table with palm up. Needle is inserted into the affected nodule and angled distally into sheath. 10 mg kenalog with 0.75 ml of 1% lidocaine (total volume 1 ml) is injected in a bolus using a 27 gauge 0.5 inch needle. Concerns include injections into tendon, hematoma and infection.

Figure credits: 14a, 14b, 14c, 14d, 14f, 14g, 14j,. Courtesy of **Cousins MJ, Bridenbaugh PO,** eds. *Neural Blockade in Clinical Anesthesia and Management of Pain,* 3rd ed. Philadelphia, Lippincott-Raven, 1998, with permission; **14e, 14i.** Courtesy of **Loeser JD, et al.,** eds. *Bonica's Management of Pain,* 3rd ed. Philadelphia, LWW, 2001, with permission.

BOTULINUM TOXIN

Botulinum toxin irreversibly blocks neuromuscular junction transmission by inhibiting pre-synaptic achetylcholine release. Botulinum toxin A (onabotulinum toxin A, Botox, Allergen), the most commonly used serotype, cleaves SNAP 25, protein needed for Ach vesicle fusion. Botox is FDA approved for strabismus, focal dystonia, hemifacial spasms, chronic migraine headaches, and for moderate to severe glabellar lines (brow furrow lines). It is also widely used off-label for spasticity and myofascial pain with favorable results. Effect onset is typically at 24–72 hours; peak effect at 2–6 weeks; clinical efficacy can last up to 3–4 months. The theoretical parenteral LD50 for a 75 kg adult is 3000 units. The recommended maximum dose is 10 units/kg IM (up to 700 units total, in practice) per visit. At least 3 months between treatments is recommended to decrease the potential for antibody formation. Botox is contraindicated in pregnancy, lactation, neuromuscular disease, concomitant aminoglycoside use, and with human albumin USP allergy. Adverse effects include pain at the injection site, weakness, nausea, and in rare cases, respiratory muscle paralysis and even death. Botox should be stored at –5 to –20° Celsius and should be reconstituted with 0.9% preservative-free saline only. Botulinum toxin B (rimabotulinum toxin B, Myobloc, Solstice) is FDA-approved for cervical dystonia. Other botulinum toxin A (Dysport, Ipsen; Xeomin, Merz) are also available in the U.S.

Suggested Botox dosing of select muscles for spasticity.

muscle	dose (U/visit) mean (range)	divided into # of sites
biceps	100 (50–100)	4
brachioradialis	50 (25–75)	2
FCR	40 (20–60)	2
FDS	20 (10–30)	1/digit
hip adductors	150 (50–250)	4
hamstrings	150 (50–250)	4
post tib	50 (25–75)	2
gastroc	50 (25–75)	2

Ch.15: SPINAL INTERVENTIONAL PROCEDURES

A. Epidural steroids

Clinical indications and efficacy - An epidural steroid injection (ESI) is typically used to alleviate neck or low back pain that is recalcitrant to more conservative measures. ESI can be especially helpful for patients during an episode of severe pain. Pain relief may also allow or enhance participation in an active rehabilitation program.

Despite the widespread use of ESIs, the medical literature has not established that ESIs are either definitely beneficial or not (Peloso, 2005; Nelemans, 2000). Many early studies and reviews, however, included patients who had had "blind" (non-fluoroscopically-guided) epidurals. The inclusion of such subjects is likely to have biased the literature towards not finding a difference between the experimental (ESI) and control groups, since "blind" epidurals frequently miss their intended targets. More recent reviews limited to ESIs delivered under fluoroscopic guidance, on the other hand, have demonstrated favorable results in groups receiving ESIs (especially for transforaminal lumbar ESIs) in comparison to controls (DePalma, 2005).

In general, patients who are likely to do well have more acute rather than chronic symptoms, and have radicular findings. Response rates are often stated to be ~80–90% when symptoms have lasted <3 mos, ~60–80% when <6 mos, and 50% or less at 1 yr or greater, although it should be noted that the rates for spontaneous resolution of pain are also not dissimilarly high. While the optimal timing for ESIs is still unknown, the early use of ESI therapy is generally advocated, rather than delaying therapy.

The interval between injections and the total number of injections allowed within a given time period are subjects of ongoing debate. While the majority of patients respond to steroids in the first few days, some may take up to a week or longer to respond. This can also depend on the type of steroid used (i.e., short-acting vs. long-acting). Moreover, there may be partial suppression of the hypothalamic-pituitary axis for about 2 wks following an ESI. It is thus often advised that repeat injections be considered after at least 2–3 wks have passed.

Generally, repeat injections may be warranted if there is partial relief of symptoms following prior injections. Because addtional relief is not well-documented after a third injection, some clinicians limit the number of ESIs to 3 injections every 6 mos or per year. In practice, the upper limit of ESIs performed in a given year to patients is highly variable, reaching as high as 20 to 40 in some academic and private practice settings according to a recent survey (Cluff, 2002). Patients not responding to the first ESI are sometimes automatically scheduled for 2nd and/or 3rd injections. There is little outcomes-based evidence in the literature supporting this empiric practice. Nonetheless, there may be a rationale to empirically repeating an ESI using a transforaminal approach if the first (ineffective) ESI was administered using an interlaminar or caudal approach.

Mechanism of action - *The mechanism of action* of ESIs is subject to debate. Proposed mechanisms include: 1) corticosteroid inhibition of phospholipase A2 released by disc injury and 2) a direct action of steroids on the spinal cord, modulating nociceptive input from peripheral nociceptors.

Contraindications and risks - *Contraindications* to ESIs include: immunocompromised states, infections, increased risk of bleeding (e.g., NSAIDs, clopidogrel, warfarin [INR >1.5], thrombocytopenia [platelets < 50K], coagulopathy), allergy to contrast or injectate, hyperglycemia, adrenal supression, and CHF. NSAIDs should be avoided for 3 days prior to procedures. Plavix and aspirin should be avoided for 7 days and Coumadin 5 days prior to procedures. Pregnancy is a contraindication to fluoroscopic procedures, although some practitioners may consider "blind" epidurals using the interlaminar approach for severe back pain. Severe central canal stenosis at the level of an injection is also a relative contraindication and the injection should be delivered slowly in this scenario. Interlaminar injections below the level of the stenosis are more desireable.

Risks of ESIs include allergic reaction, complications of steroids (e.g., fluid retention, facial flushing, hyperglycemia, euphoria), infection, epidural bleed, thecal puncture, and spinal cord injury (unlikely). Particulate steroids inadvertently injected into the vasculature have been implicated in central nervous system infarcts (Derby, 2008). Intrathecal steroid administration has been associated with anterior spinal artery syndrome, arachnoiditis, and conus medullaris syndrome, and is best avoided. However, intrathecal steroids have been successfully used to treat intractable post-herpetic neuralgia without report of significant complication (Kotani, 2000).

Ref: **Peloso P, et al.** Medicinal and injection therapies for mechanical neck disorders. *Cochrane Database Syst Rev* 2005;(2):CD000319; **Nelemans PJ, et al.** Injection therapy for subacute and chronic benign LBP. *Cochrane Database Syst Rev* 2000;(2):CD001824; **DePalma MJ, et al.** A critical appraisal of the evidence for selective nerve root injection in the tx of lumbosacral radiculopathy. *Arch Phys Med Rehab* 2005;86:1477; **Cluff R, et al.** The technical aspects of epidural steroid injections: a national survey. *Anesth Analg* 2002;95:403; **Derby R, et al.** Size and aggregation of corticosteroids used for epidural injections. *Pain Med* 2008;(9):227; **Kotani N, et al.** Intrathecal methylprednisolone for intractable postherpetic neuralgia. *NEJM* 2000;343:1514.

Technical considerations

The use of fluoroscopy is now strongly recommended to confirm proper needle placement in the epidural space, as it is missed with high frequency in "blind" epidurals, even in experienced hands (25–30% miss rate for lumbosacral ESIs [White, 1980], and higher in cervical ESIs). In addition, the use of contrast media is recommended to confirm placement, and also because negative aspirations for blood can be falsely negative.

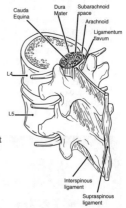

Figure 15a1 Relevant anatomy for the interlaminar approach.

The *interlaminar ESI* (ILESI, also known as translaminar ESI) can take a midline or paramedian path. In the midline approach, the needle traverses through the thick interspinous ligament until it penetrates the ligamentum flavum (often a "pop" is felt) and is in the epidural space. The paramedian approach (~10–15° off the midline) avoids the interspinous ligament and traverses through the paraspinal muscles and ligamentum flavum. An ILESI is not indicated for patients who has had laminectomy, due to the absence of the ligamentum flavum.

The ILESI is performed at the clinically symptomatic level. In the cervical spine, a typical injectate may be 3–5 ml of 40–60 mg of methylprednisolone mixed in 1–2% lidocaine or saline. In the lumbar spine, a typical injectate may be 6–10 ml of 80–120 mg of methylprednisolone mixed in 1–2% lidocaine or saline.

Autopsy studies have shown that the spinal cord extends caudally no further than L2 for the majority of the population (see figure 15a2). The risk of spinal cord injury due to direct trauma during interlaminar injections is very low, but not non-existent above this level.

The **transforaminal ESI** (TFESI, aka periradicular injection) delivers the injectate more anteriorly than the ILESI, targeting the nerve root. TFESIs are appropriate for patients with post-laminectomy syndrome. Targeting treatment to right and/or left sides at one or multiple levels is possible. TFESIs are particularly effective for far lateral disc herniations affecting specific nerve roots, since the pathological area can be directly addressed. ILESIs, in contrast, depend on diffusion of the injectate, which may not occur sufficiently enough for clinical relief.

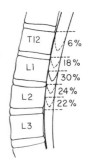

Figure 15a2 Caudal extent of the spinal cord.

The lumbar TFESI is performed with the C-arm rotated to reveal an oblique view of the spine. Once the "Scotty dog" view is obtained, the C-arm is adjusted until the superior articular process (the ear of the "Scotty dog") is halfway between the anterior and posterior portion of the vertebral body superior end plate. The superior end plate of the vertebral body should appear superimposed on fluoroscopy. The nerve root passes a few mm inferior to the pedicle and 1–2 mm superficial to the vertebral body. The needle is advanced toward the superior aspect of the neuroforamen, just inferior to the pedicle. With the C-arm rotated to a lateral view, needle is further advanced until the tip is in the dorsal and cephalad quadrant of the neuroforamen, taking care to withdraw the needle slightly if paresthesia is encountered. After a negative aspiration, a small amount of contrast media should be injected to confirm epidural spread and to detect intravascular uptake. Less injectate is used than for ILESIs (about half or less of the interlaminar amounts). Special care, however, should be taken to avoid injection into the artery of Adamkiewicz (which enters the spinal canal in the lower thoracic or lumbar spinal levels near the nerve root), as this can result in a spinal cord infarct.

Cervical TFESIs confer the advantage of reducing cephalad spread (sometimes seen with ILESIs, leading to respiratory depression), but are somewhat controversial due to the risk of substantial adverse events (e.g., vascular injection, tetraplegia, hemiplegia), even if they occur only infrequently.

TFESIs are often interchangeably used with selective nerve root blocks (SNRB), although the latter usually refers to injections done to affect a single nerve root without the injectate necessarily reaching the epidural space.

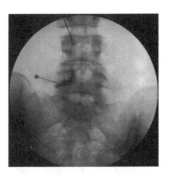
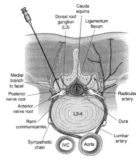

Figure 15a3 TFESI, AP fluoroscopic view (left) and schematic (right).

A *caudal ESI* can be considered if a lumbar TFESI or ILESI approach is technically difficult. Although caudals are sometimes given for coccydynia, the efficacy for this is unclear. Larger injectate volumes (e.g., 20 ml) are typically used and specific spinal structures not targeted. Thecal puncture risk is lowest with caudals since the thecal sac typically ends at or above S2. Sacral abscess is a known but very unlikely complication.

Local anesthetic is usually given in the area of the sacral cornu, which is easily palpated. A spinal needle with injectate is placed just inferior to the sacral cornu and advanced using fluoroscopic guidance. Contrast dye should be used to observe flow of the injectate to the lower lumbar levels with lateral and A-P views. The injectate will flow in a predominantly cephalad direction toward the lower lumbar levels.

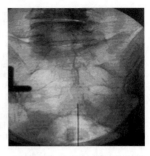

Figure 15a4 Caudal ESI. The needle is in the epidural space.

Ref: White AJ, et al. Epidural injections for the dx and tx of LBP. *Spine* 1980;5:78; **Renfrew DL.** Correct placement of epidural steroid injections: fluoroscopic guidance and contrast administration. *AJNR* 1991;12:1003; **Rydevik B.** Pathoanatomy and pathophysiology of nerve root compression. *Spine* 1984;9:7. **Figure credits: 15a1, 15a2.** Courtesy of **Loeser JD, et al.**, eds. *Bonica's Management of Pain*, 3rd ed. Philadelphia, LWW, 2001, with permission; **15a3.** Radiograph courtesy of **Ballantyne JC.** *The MGH Handbook of Pain Management*, 3rd ed. Philadelphia, LWW, 2006, with permission. Schematic courtesy of **Rathmell JP.** *Atlas of imaging in regional anesthesia and pain medicine.* Philadelphia, LWW, 2005, modified with permission.

B. Zygapophysial (facet) joint injections and RF neurotomy

Anatomy - The zygapophysial joint is also known as the z-joint or facet joint, although use of the latter term is being discouraged. Z-joints are true diarthrodial joints with hyaline cartilage, synovial membranes, and fibrous capsules. The fibrous capsules contain mechanoreceptors and nociceptors, while the subsynovial tissues contain nociceptors. These nociceptors arise from the sympathetic and parasympathetic ganglia.

In the cervical spine, the C2–C3 joint is innervated by two branches of the dorsal ramus of the third cervical nerve: a communicating branch and a medial branch known as the third occipital nerve. Below that in the cervical spine, the innervation of each joint comes from the medial branches of the dorsal rami from each spinal nerve above and below the joint; e.g., the medial branches of C3 and C4 innervate the C3–4 facet. In the lumbar spine, each z-joint is innervated by the medial branch of the dorsal ramus of the spinal nerve at the same level as well as the medial branch from one level rostrally (e.g., the L4–5 z-joint is innervated by medial branches from L3 and L4), with the exception of the L5-S1 z-joint, which in addition to L4 and L5 medial branch nerves may receive additional innervation from S1 medial branch nerve ("triple-innervated").

Clinical evaluation and efficacy of the interventional therapies - Z-joint pain cannot easily be diagnosed by history, physical exam, or imaging. Historical elements supportive of z-joint pain include pain that worsens with extension (e.g., when standing from a seated position). The exam may be notable for a positive "facet loading maneuver," but the straight leg raise test is usually negative. Diagnostic blocks of the z-joints or nerves supplying the joints under fluoroscopic guidance are the only means available to firmly establish the z-joints as pain generators. A small volume injection is necessary to maximize diagnostic integrity. A typical volume for a diagnostic medial branch block is 0.5–1 ml.

If conservative management is unsuccessful, therapeutic injections intraarticularly or near the nervous supply can be considered. Intraarticular steroids and/or local anesthetics can alleviate joint inflammation and wash away potential chemical irritants. A normal joint will accommodate 1.0–1.5 ml of injectate. Some favor only treating the medial branches to avoid potential damage to the joint. Radiofrequency ablation of the innervation is another option. High-grade evidence in the medical literature supporting these interventions, however, is still scant. The quality of the methods and designs of many studies in the literature has been poor, with high variability in the diagnostic criteria and variations in definition of a successful outcome.

Contraindications to z-joint intraarticular injection include INR >1.5, allergies to injectate, active systemic infection or skin lesions, malignancy, recent surgery, and pregnancy (secondary to the need for fluorscopic exposure).

Technique - For cervical z-joint medial branch injections, the patient is placed in the lateral position. For cervical intraarticular injections, it is more difficult to gain joint access from a lateral approach so a posterior approach should be considered. A 25-gauge 1.5 inch needle is used for cervical z-joint and medial branch injections. Care must be exercised to prevent injury to local vascular structures. Use of contrast is adviseable to ensure the needle is in the proper position and to minimize the potential for vascular injection. The C3–7 z-joints are innervated by medial branches that run along the articular pillar in the cervical spine, varying in height and position along the vertebral body. The C2–3 joint is unique as the needle should be placed just lateral to the joint at the location of the large third occipital nerve that innervates the joint. Knowledge of the local anatomy is essential to the performance of these procedures.

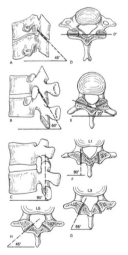

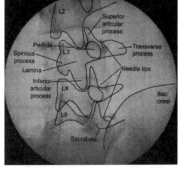

Figure 15b1 Z-joint angles in C-Spine, T-spine and L-spine.

Figure 15b2 Lumbar Z-joint injections (fluoroscopic view)

For lumbar z-joint injections, the patient is placed in the prone position. A 22 or 25-gauge 3.5 inch spinal needle is most often used. The ideal entry point for intraarticular injections is at the inferolateral edge of the inferior articulating process, as this is the largest area for injection. From L1–4, the medial branch lies at the intersection of the superior articular process and transverse process. Since the transverse process of S1 is replaced by the sacral ala, L5 'medial branch block' is actually performed as L5 dorsal ramus block, the target being the junction between the sacral ala and the superior articular process.

Radiofrequency (RF) neurotomy/ ablation - RF is a high frequency current that generates a well circumscribed spheroidal lesion and thermocoagulates target neural tissue. (Use of the term "rhizotomy" is discouraged, since this refers to cutting a nerve.) RF ablation of the dorsal medial branch (to block all sensory input from the joint) has long been advocated for recalcitrant z-joint pain which has been confirmed with one or more diagnostic blocks. If the z-joint is the primary pain generator for a given patient, symptomatic relief can be expected by denervating the nervous supply to the z-joint. Pain frequently recurs, however, once the medial branch axons regenerate. Larger lesions can reduce recurrence of pain, but also risk excessive local damage, including non-target neural tissue. Local temperature at the electrode tip should be monitored to create safe and predictable lesions. Temperature >90° Celsius will cause tissue to boil and should be avoided. Sensory and motor stimulation prior to RF lesioning is helpful to avoid injury to the motor nerves. Pulsed RF has been proposed as a way to perform RF at lower temperature and without permanent nerve injury.

Overall, the published outcomes for z-joint RF ablation is equivocal. A 2003 Cochrane review revealed limited evidence that RF denervation offers short-term relief for chronic neck pain of z-joint origin and for chronic cervicobrachial pain, and conflicting evidence for its effectiveness for lumbar z-joint pain. Design issues in the research published to date has precluded definitive conclusions. Some recent reviews have questioned the efficacy of radiofrequency neurotomy in treating z-joint mediated pain (Carragee, 2008; Chou, 2009).

Generally, patients carefully selected on the basis of differential dorsal medial branch diagnostic blocks (>80% relief for >1 hr with lidocaine and >2 hrs with bupivacaine) are the best candidates for denervation procedures (Dreyfuss, 2000).

Ref: **Carragee EJ, et al.** Treatment of neck pain: injections and surgical interventions: results of the Bone and Joint Decade 2000–2010 Task Force on Neck Pain and Its Associated Disorders. *Spine* 2008;15:S153. **Chou R, et al.** Nonsurgical interventional therapies for low back pain: a review of the evidence for an American Pain Society clinical practice guideline. *Spine* 2009;34:1078; **Niemisto L, et al.** Radiofrequency denervation for neck and back pain: a systematic review within the framework of the Cochrane collaboration back review group. *Spine* 2003;28:1877; **Dreyfuss P, et al.** Efficacy and validity of radiofrequency neurotomy for chronic lumbar zygapophysial joint pain. *Spine* 2000;25:1270. **Figure credits: 15b1.** Courtesy of Loeser JD, et al., eds. *Bonica's Management of Pain*, 3rd ed. Philadelphia, LWW, 2001, with permission; **15b2.** Schematic courtesy of **Rathmell JP.** *Atlas of imaging in regional anesthesia and pain medicine.* Philadelphia, LWW, 2005, with permission. Radiograph courtesy of **Ballantyne JC.** *The MGH Handbook of Pain Management*, 3rd ed. Philadelphia, LWW, 2006, with permission.

C. Sacroiliac joint (SIJ) injection

Epidemiology - The sacroiliac joint (SIJ) was thought to be primary cause of low back pain until a hallmark article by Mixter and Barr (1934), which presented the herniated disc as a source of low back pain. Presently, the prevalence of SIJ-related pain is unclear, but it is thought to be underdiagnosed. The etiologies for the SIJ syndrome are many, but the majority of cases are due to a traumatic event (44%) such as MVA or fall (typically a direct fall on the buttocks) or are idiopathic (35%; Chou, 2004).

Anatomy and clinical evaluation - The SIJ is a true diarthrodial joint with hyaline and fibrocartilage. Controversies related to the innervation of the joint abound, but a recent review of the anatomical literature suggests that the SIJ is innervated by the sacral dorsal rami (Forst, 2006). Nerve fibers penetrate the adjoining ligaments and joint capsule.

Pain typically refers to the gluteus and thigh but can also reach the groin or calf. Positive findings on provocative tests such as Gaenslen's, Patrick's, Yeoman's and Gillet's may aid in the diagnosis of SIJ syndrome, although the validitiy of the tests has been questioned (Dreyfuss, 1994).

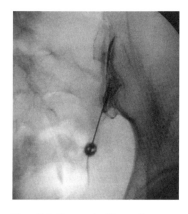

Figure 15c1 Fluoroscopic still image of contrast dye outlining sacroiliac joint.

Criteria per the International Association for the Study of Pain for SIJ syndrome include: 1) pain in the region of the SIJ, with possible radiation to the groin, medial buttocks, and posterior thigh; 2) reproduction of pain by physical examination techniques that stress the joint; 3) elimination of pain with intraarticular injection of local anesthetic; and 4) ostensibly morphologically normal joint w/o other demonstrable pathognomonic radiographic abnormality.

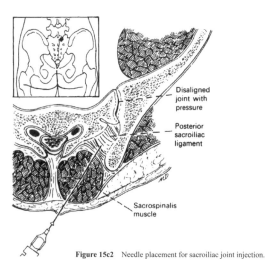

Disaligned joint with pressure

Posterior sacroiliac ligament

Sacrospinalis muscle

Figure 15c2 Needle placement for sacroiliac joint injection.

Because SIJ pain can mimic lumbar radiculopathy or facet-mediated pain, ruling out these conditions is needed for the accurate diagnosis of SIJ pain.

Technique - The patient is placed in the prone postion. The C-arm is in an oblique position. The inferior one-third of the SIJ is identified with fluoroscopy. The margins of the anterior and posterior joint lines are aligned such that they overlap.

A long needle (e.g., 22-gauge 3.5 inch spinal needle) is directed to the inferior 1/3 of the joint. After aspiration (to confirm a non-intravascular position), injection of contrast is performed to assess joint flow. Injection of 2–3 ml of local anesthetic (e.g., 1% lidocaine) and corticosteroid (optional) is placed.

Ref: Mixter WJ, Barr JS. Rupture of the intervertebral disc with involvement of the spinal canal. *NEJM* 1934;211:210; **Chou LH.** Inciting events initiating injection-proven sacroiliac joint syndrome. *Pain Med* 2004;5:26; **Forst SL, et al.** The SIJ: anatomy, physiology and clinical significance. *Pain Physician* 2006;9:61; **Dreyfuss P.** Positive sacroiliac screening tests in asymptomatic adults. *Spine* 1994;19:1138;
Figure credits: 15c2. Courtesy of **Loeser JD, et al., eds.** *Bonica's Management of Pain, 3rd ed.* Philadelphia, LWW, 2001, with permission.

D. Stellate ganglion block

Indication: Diagnosis of sympathetically mediated pain, including complex regional pain syndrome (CRPS), of the upper extremity. Possible utility as a predictor prior to a spinal cord stimulator trial.

Anatomy: The stellate ganglion is formed by the fusion of the inferior cervical and first thoracic sympathetic ganglia. It is ~2 cm long, lies in the C7-T1 interspace, anterior to the head of the first rib and longus colli muscle.

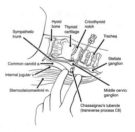

Technique: The *anterior paratracheal approach* involves placement of the needle at the medial edge of the sternocleidomastoid (SCM) at the level of the cricothyroid and C6. With the patient supine, the needle is inserted medial to the carotid arteries at the C6 transverse process, then withdrawn 2–5 mm. It is generally the safest and least painful technique. Other approaches include *posterior approach* and *vertebral body approach* placing the needle at the junction of the transverse process and vertebral body of C7. Traditionally, SGBs have been performed by blind technique. Lately, fluoroscopic and CT-guided techniques have become more commonly used, allowing for the more targeted delivery of a smaller volume of injectate (3–5 ml vs. ≥10 ml for blind techniques) and reducing the likelihood of adverse effects.

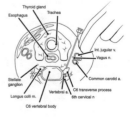

Adverse effects: A temporary ipsilateral Horner's syndrome (ptosis, miosis, anhydrosis, scleral injection, nasal congestion) is expected and confirms a proper injection. An increase of ipsilateral more than contralateral skin temperatures at the distal hand also is

Figure 15d Anterior paratracheal approach for SGB.

confirmatory. Complications of SGBs include: permanent Horner's syndrome, recurrent laryngeal nerve injury (voice hoarseness), dysphagia, phrenic nerve injury (paralyzed hemidiaphragm), brachial plexus block, epidural block, pneumothorax, seizure due to inadvertent vascular injection, and retropharyngeal hematoma (rare but can be fatal).

E. Lumbar sympathetic block

Indication: Diagnosis of sympathetically mediated pain, including complex regional pain syndrome (CRPS), of the lower extremity. Possible utility as a predictor prior to a spinal cord stimulator trial.

Anatomy: Lumbar sympathetic chain consists of several ganglia that run along both sides of the vertebral body. The ganglia are most commonly found between lower border of L2 to middle region of L3. Psoas muscle is posterior to the sympathetic chain and separates the sympathetic chain from the somatic nerve roots, minimizing side effects from spread of injectate.

Technique: Patient is placed prone. Fluoroscopy machine identifies L2 vertebral body in AP view. Location ~7 cm lateral from midline is demarcated. Using intermittent biplar fluoroscopy, a 22-gauge 5-inch needle is advanced until it contacts the L2 vertebral body. The needle is then walked off until the needle tip lies at the anterolateral border of the L2 vertebral body. After aspiration reveals negative heme or CSF, 1–3 ml of contrast is used to confirm the characteristic longitudinal pattern of the contrast dye. A test dose of 2 ml of local anesthetic is injected to evaluate for untoward side effect. About 5–8 ml of local anesthetic is then injected. The procedure may then be repeated at L3 level.

Adverse effects: Pain at the site of injection. Somatic nerve block with inadvertent injection into psoas muscle. Puncture of the kidney or ureter. Puncture of peritoneal cavity. Perforation of the aorta or IVC. Genitofemoral nerve block. Retroperitoneal hemorrhage. Epidural or subarachnoid block.

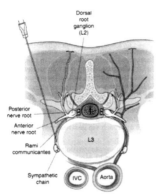

Figure 15e Lumbar parasympathetic block. Figure courtesy of Rathmell JP. *Atlas of imaging in regional anesthesia and pain medicine.* Philadelphia, LWW, 2005.

F. Celiac plexus block

Indication: Pancreatic ca, chronic pancreatitis.

Anatomy: Greater, lesser, and least splanchnic nerves synapse with celiac ganglion, which send fibers to celiac plexus. Celiac plexus (mix of sympathetic and visceral afferent innervation) lie in the anterocrural (front of diaphragm) space in front of L1 vertebral body around celiac artery.

Techniques:

1. *retrocrural approach:* with patient prone, find T12 spinous process, go 7 cm lateral, introduce needle aiming slightly inferior so it would contact L1 vertebral body, walk off to postion needle just in front of the vertebral body (not to go past 1–2 cm in front of vertebral body); perform injection on both sides (requires two needles). Inject 12–25 ml of local anesthetic.

2. *transcrural approach:* similar to retrocrural approach, except that the needle is advanced to the crura, then advanced slightly further until the needle tip lies anterior to the crura; slightly smaller volume of injectate needed than the retrocrural approach; requires injection on both sides (2 needles).

3. *transaortic approach:* with patient prone, introduce single needle on left; possible lower incidence of complications (no retrocrural spread, hence potentially less possibility of neurologic sequelae), concern for dislodging atherosclerotic plaque in elderly, dosage = 10–15 ml local anesthetic (Ischia, 1983).

4. *anterior approach:* with patient supine, fine needle (32 gauge) is introduced into celiac plexus; requires needle going through liver, stomach, intestine, vasculature, and pancreas; potential lower incidence of complications (Montero Matamala, 1988); risk of infection, abscess, hemorrhage, fistula formation.

Side effects: Hypotension (administer IV fluid [1 L] before procedure); diarrhea.

Complication: Potential for lower extremity paralysis.

Ref: Ischia S, et al. A new approach to the neurolytic block of the coeliac plexus: the transaortic technique. *Pain* 1983;16:333; **Feldstein GS, et al.** Loss of resistance technique for transaortic celiac plexus block. *Anesth Analg* 1986;65:1092; **Montero Matamala A, et al.** The percutaneous anterior approach to the celiac plexus using CT guidance. *Pain* 1988;34:285.

G. Superior hypogastric plexus block

Indication: Pelvic pain secondary to malignant and nonmalignant pain. Superior hypogastric plexus receives visceral sensory afferent traffic within the pelvis. Any visceral afferent signal from pelvis is relayed via superior hypogastric plexus. Generally lies anterior to L5/S1 vertebral bodies.

Technique: Similar to discography at L5/S1; can be technically challenging. Patient is positioned prone. Spinal needle enters 7 cm from midline at L4 level and directed inferiorly to contact L5 vertebral body, at which point needle is directed further inferiorly. After position is confirmed with 3–5 ml of contrast under fluoroscopy, 6–10 ml of local anesthetic (or phenol if neurolysis) is injected. The procedure is then repeated on the contralateral side.

Complications: Hematoma, injection site pain, somatic block from subarachnoid or epidural injection, somatic nerve injury, ureteral/renal puncture. Avoid bilateral block in men secondary to possibility of sexual dysfunction (Sayson, 2004).

Sayson SC and Ramamurthy S. Sympathetic Blocks. in: Warfield CA and Bajwa, ZH, eds. *Principles and Practice of Pain Medicine*. New York, NY: McGraw-Hill; 2004:703.

H. Ganglion Impar block

Ganglion of Walther is a solitary terminal ganglion of sympathetic chains located anterior to sacrococcygeal junction.

Indication: Intractable perineal pain secondary to rectal/bladder/cervical cancer.

Classic method: Needle bent 90 degrees, introduce needle beneath the coccyx. Inject 4–6 ml of local anesthetic or neurolytic agent.

Midline method: Obtain lateral view, introduce needle through the ligament between sacrum and coccyx, ascertain contrast spread, inject 4–6 ml local anesthetic or neurolytic agent.

Complications: Bowel perforation, injection side pain.

I. Subarachnoid neurolysis with alcohol and phenol

Indication: Intractable pain from malignancy. Goal is for sensory blockade while minimizing motor weakness.

Alcohol is hypobaric, postion patient in lateral decub with affected side up (useful for patients who cannot lie on affected side); burning on injection confirms diagnosis; inject 0.1 mL incrementally; use 0.7 mL max per spinal nerve root.

Phenol is hyperbaric, will tend to sink in the intrathecal space; position patient so that the patient is lateral decub with affected area down.

J. Intradiscal electrothermic annuloplasty (IDEA)

Intradiscal electrothermic annuloplasty (IDEA) is an FDA-approved (1998) option for treating discogenic spinal pain. Note that Intradiscal Electrothermic Therapy (IDET) is a trademarked term.

Following disc injuries, nerve endings can grow from their normal location in the annulus to inside the nucleus, or nuclear material can enter the annulus and irritate the annular nociceptors. IDEA's putative mechanism of action in relieving discogenic pain is the destruction of nociceptors in the disc by thermal modification. The disc is essentially desensitized.

As is the case for many procedures for LBP, e.g., fusion, there are few high-quality studies examining the clinical efficacy of IDEA to date. An early case-control series by Bogduk's group (2000) reported that patients receiving IDEA had reduced pain, analgesic usage, and disability, as well as increased return to work rates in comparison to a convenience sample undergoing conservative rehabilitation. The effects lasted at least one year. A retrospective survey of 44 patients showed low patient satisfaction rates (37%), high rates of persistent pain (97%), and no significant difference in disability status at one year following IDEA (Davis, 2004). A recent randomized, controlled trial failed to demonstrate significant positive outcomes in pain and function at 6 months following IDEA vs. sham procedure (Freeman, 2005). With continued technique refinement and strict adherence to appropriate patient selection, however, the success rate following IDEA may rise.

Patient selection and outcome predictors - A trial of conservative therapy over at least 6 months is indicated prior to an IDEA trial. Ideal candidates for IDEA have only one or two disc level involvement, preserved disc heights (>50%), and do not have a severe radicular component to their pain. Patients should also be able to commit to substantial post-procedural activity restrictions.

A pre-procedural discogram should show only limited tears, with a generally healthy disc annulus. Pressure measurements should show a highly irritated, sensitive disc, i.e., similar pains should be elicited at low injection pressures. If the discogram shows severe pathology or an insensitive disc with no tears, IDEA may not be warranted.

Poor outcome predictors include provider self-referral for IDEA and a history of significant opioid use (Webster, 2004). Discal healing may be compromised in older patients, reducing the likelihood of positive outcomes.

Absolute contraindications include disc herniation, significant spinal instability (e.g., spondylolysis or spondylolisthesis), spinal stenosis, and severe disc anatomical degeneration.

Relative contraindications include previously surgically-treated discs, and severe or multilevel discogenic pain.

Procedure - Patients should be NPO, except for water, 4 hrs prior to IDEA. The patient's usual meds should be continued on the day of the procedure, except for anti-inflammatories or other blood thinners such as coumadin or clopidogrel, which must be discontinued 4 days prior to IDEA. Sedatives and local anesthetics are given right before IDEA.

A hollow introducer needle is placed into the problematic disc(s) under fluoroscopy. A flexible catheter and heating element are threaded through the introducer until the catheter sits circumferentially along the inner surface of the annulus, with the tip through the tear(s). The heating element is then turned on, with a target temperature of 80–90° C for ~5 mins. Any nerve fibers exposed to the high levels of heat are destroyed. To minimize discitis, local antibiotics are given at each disc level. After the procedure, as the heated areas cool, the disc tissue stiffens and "toughens," effectively repairing annular tears. Immediately after IDEA, oral or IV pain meds can be given.

Pain will normally increase mildly for a few days to weeks. To promote maximum discal healing, no lifting of heavy loads or aggressive physical activity is allowed for at least 6 months. In fact, only minimal movement at the treated levels is advised. For example, there should be limited bending and twisting of the treated levels of the spine, limited periods of sitting upright, and only light walking until physical therapy is started (usually at ~6–12 wks post-IDEA).

Potential complications of IDEA include discitis, disc damage, bleeding, and nerve injury including spinal cord injury.

Refs: Karasek M, Bogduk N. Twelve-month follow-up of a controlled trial of intradiscal thermal annuloplasty for back pain due to internal disc disruption. *Spine* 2000;25:2601; **Davis TT, et al.** The IDET procedure for chronic discogenic LBP. *Spine* 2004;29:752; **Freeman BJ, et al.** A randomized, double-blind, controlled trial: IDET vs. placebo for the treatment of chronic discogenic LBP. *Spine* 2005;30:2369; **Webster BS, et al.** Outcomes of workers' compensation claimants with low back pain undergoing intradiscal electrothermal therapy. *Spine* 2004;29:435.

K. Percutaneous disc decompression

Percutaneous disc decompression is used for spinal pain with a radicular component caused by a disc protrusion. Decompression at the disc center is thought to reduce the peripheral herniation. Techniques include mechanical disc removal, chemonucleolysis, laser decompression, and nucleoplasty using radiofrequency waves.

Percutaneous disc decompression via **chemonucleolysis** has been around for a long time, first performed in the 1960s. This procedure involves the chemical dissolution of nucleus pulposus via a percutaneous injection into the nucleus, most commonly using chymopapain, a proteolytic enzyme derived from the papaya fruit. This enzyme cleaves the proteoglycan into substituent mucoprotein and glycosaminoglycan. Unfortunately, the procedure has been associated with a number of problems that have limited its use. First, it is difficult to predict the amount of nucleus that will be digested, leading to cases of over-decompression, disc collapse, and instability. Chymopapain is indiscriminate in the proteins that it will digest, and it may cause neural damage if it comes into contact with neural elements. There have been a number of rare, though serious, complications associated with chemonucleolysis. In addition, there is an estimated 0.5% incidence of anaphylactic reactions to this enzyme, leading to a number of deaths. Because of these complications, use of chemonucleolysis has decreased significantly.

Percutaneous laser discectomy - Choy et al. introduced the YAG laser to vaporize nucleus pulposus in 1991. In a large series of patients treated over many years, the overall success rate was reported as greater than 75 percent. Concerns have been raised regarding the thermal energy transfer during laser discectomy. There can be a significant rise in temperature throughout the disc, including at the endplate and nerve root. These higher temperatures often result in significant postoperative pain and spasm, which has made this procedure less popular.

Nucleoplasty utilizes a percutaneous approach to decompress disc material. This is accomplished via a multifunctional bipolar radiofrequency device that features Coblation technology to ablate, or remove tissue, while alternating with thermal energy for coagulation. Because these effects are achieved at temperatures of approximately 40–70°C, thermal damage to surrounding tissue is minimized.

Nucleoplasty is performed on an outpatient basis. Fluoroscopic imaging is used to facilitate percutaneous placement of an introducer needle at the nucleus/annulus junction. The SpineWand is introduced through an introducer needle and advanced into the nucleus using ablation mode. Channeling is stopped prior to reaching the anterior annular wall. Coagulation mode is then used while withdrawing the Wand at approximately 0.5 cm/second. The same procedure is repeated six times within the disc. After the needle is removed, bandage is applied on the skin and the patient is discharged home. Patients are then placed on a routine rehabilitation program as part of the standard protocol for interventional spinal procedures. Complications are rare and similar to those associated with discography.

Automated Percutaneous Lumbar Discectomy - Hijikata first described the manual percutaneous decompression of nucleus pulposus in 1975, utilizing a fenestrated punch. In 1985, Onik and his coworkers developed a blunt-tipped, reciprocating, suction-cutting probe for automated percutaneous lumbar discectomy (APLD). Manchikanti et al. (2009) in a comprehensive review deemed APLD to have II-2 level (evidence obtained from at least one properly designed small diagnostic accuracy study) of evidence for efficacy.

Refs: **Hijikata S.** Percutaneous nucleotomy. A new concept technique and 12 years' experience. *Clinical Ortho* 1989;9:238; **Choy DS, et al.** Percutaneous laser disc decompression. A new therapeutic modality. *Spine* 1992;17:949; **Manchitanki L, et al.** Comprehensive evidence-based guidelines for interventional techniques in the management of chronic spinal pain. *Pain Physician* 2009;12:699.

L. Vertebroplasty and kyphoplasty

Vertebroplasty is used in the management of pain from vertebral compression fractures. The first published use of percutaneous vertebroplasty with methylmethacrylate was by Galibert et al. in 1990. The mechanism of pain relief is believed to be mechanical stabilization of the fracture via stabilization of vertebral bodies and offloading of the z-joints. There may also be analgesia from local chemical, vascular, or thermal effects from PMMA (polymethyl-methacrylate) on nerve endings. Restoration of height is also thought to improve the biomechanics of spine.

Plain frontal and lateral radiographs are the initial imaging studies. Positive compression fracture is typified by a radiographic evidence of decrease in vertebral height of 20% or more, or a decrease of at least 4 mm from baseline.

Compression fractures can occur anywhere from the occiput to the sacrum, but the usual sites are T8–T12, L1, and L4.

The more recent the fracture, the greater likelihood the procedure will be effective (fractures <2 years old), and pain at the level or within one vertebral body up/down from the fracture offer better outcome.

Some have questioned the efficacy of vertebroplasty. A pair of randomized sham-procedure controlled trials have indicated that improvement in pain is similar between those treated with vertebroplasty and those in the control group (Buchbinder, 2009; Kallmes, 2009).

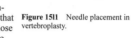

Figure 15l1 Needle placement in vertebroplasty.

Contraindications include fractures with >80% loss of height; fractures with retropulsed fragment or lytic involvement of the posterior cortex (injection of cement can cause further migration of fragment); poorly localized pain or pain that does not correlate with level of fracture; systemic or local active infection, especially the skin overlying the site; or the patient unable to lie prone for 30 to 45 minutes.

The vertebral body can be targeted by different approaches. There is a *trans-pedicular approach* for the thoracolumbar spine, and an *anterolateral approach* for the cervical spine.

Complications include cement extrava-sation, which increases with osteolytic fractures; PMMA with liquid rather than pasty consistency; or higher PMMA vol-ume. Depending on location, extravasation can lead to more serious consequences, including epidural/foraminal nerve root compression and pulmonary embolism via the perivertebral veins. Extravasation into adjacent discs or paravertebral tissues is generally asymptomatic.

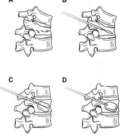

Figure 15l2 Use of balloon in kyphoplasty.

Kyphoplasty is similar to vertebroplasty, except for the use of a balloon to help expand the volume of the fractured segment prior to introducing the cement polymer. Potentially, it leads to a better correction of the deformity (i.e., better restoration of vertebral height). The risk of cement extravasation is believed to be reduced due to higher cement viscosity and lower pressure during the injection.

Procedure consists of the balloon being placed coaxially through a needle into the vertebral body to reduce the fracture, followed by introduction of cement. Kyphoplasty requires larger (9–10 gauge) needles and a bipedicular approach, hence, limiting the targeted areas to thoracic and lumbar levels. Injection via transpedicular or paravertbral approach is performed under continuous fluoroscopic guidance.

Refs: Galibert P, et al. Note preliminaire sur le traitement des angiomes vertebraux et des affections dolorigenes et fragilisantes du rachis, *Chirurgie* 1990;116:326; **Buchbinder R, et al.** A Randomized Trial of Vertebroplasty for Painful Osteoporotic Vertebral Fractures. *NEJM* 2009;361:557; **Kallmes DF, et al.** A Randomized Trial of Vertebroplasty for Osteoporotic Spinal Fractures. *NEJM* 2009;361:569; **Lieberman I and Reinhardt MK.** Vertebroplasty and

Kyphoplasty for Osteolytic Vertebral Collapse, *Clinical Orthopedics and Related Research*, 415S: pp. S176. **Fenton D and Czervionke L.** Image Guided Spine Intervention. W.B. Saunders Company (2002). p 189.

M. Intrathecal pump

The direct administration of opioids near spinal cord receptors is an effective modality for pain control. Yaksh (1976) demonstrated that intraspinal opioids modulate pain by inhibitory mechanisms at the spinal cord. Wang (1979) reported excellent results with the use of intrathecal morphine for cancer pain. An externally programmable, fully implantable pump was first introduced in 1988. The pump can be filled with various medications including opioids, clonidine, baclofen, bupivicaine, and ziconotide (Rainov, 2001).

Indications for intrathecal pump implantation include the need for intrathecal opioids in cancer pain or chronic nonmalignant pain in patients who do not tolerate oral medications, and those needing intrathecal baclofen for spasticity.

Absolute contraindications include aplastic anemia, systemic infection, known allergies to the implant material or to the intended medication, active IV drug use, psychosis or dementia. *Relative contraindications* include emaciation, ongoing anticoagulation therapy, young age (before fusion of epiphyses), possible occult infection, recovering drug addict, lack of access to medical care, lack of social/family support, socioeconomic problem, and non-response to opioids. Olson (1992) identified more risk factors for poor outcome with implantable opioid therapy, such as mood disorder, potential for self-harm, anxiety, high magnitude of stress including catastrophizing, addictive issues, and sleep disturbances.

Complications of intrathecal pumps include infections, surgical/device-related problems (catheter problems most common), and complications from the drug (e.g., overdosage). Catheter kinking, mechanical failure, catheter tip granulomas and infections can occur. Significant neurological, urological and respiratory symptoms can occur and result in adverse consequences such as urinary retention and respiratory suppression. Less significant side effects such as decreased libido, pruritus, peripheral edema, and constipation are more common (Paice 1997). In one study involving 97 patients, 44% patients reported various complications, the most common being pharmacological side effects (34%), equipment (16%), programming (2%), catheter (6%), and infection (1%) (Kamran, 2001).

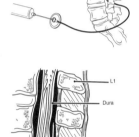

Figure 15m1 Shown is a needle with medication being introduced into the pump via the pump portal. The medication is delivered into the intrathecal space via the catheter. Catheter is shown threaded intrathecally via the L3/4 interlaminar space.

Ref: **Oakley J and Staats PS.** In Raj PP, ed. Practical Management of Pain, 3rd ed. Mosby, St. Louis, 2000. Chapter 54: The Use of Implanted Drug Delivery Systems, p 768–778. **Rainov NG,**

et al. Long-Term Intrathecal Infusion of Drug Combinations for Chronic Back and Leg Pain. *J Pain Symptom Management* 2001;22:862; **Olson K.** An Approach to Psychological Assessment of Chronic Pain Patients. Minneapolis, NCS Assessments, 1992. **Wang JK et al.** Pain relief by intrathecally applied morphine in pain. *Anesthesiology* 1979;50:149; **Yaksh TL, Rudy T.** Analgesia mediated by a direct spinal action of narcotics. *Science* 1976;192:1357; **Paice JA, et al.** Clinical Realities and Economic Considerations: Efficacy of Intrathecal Pain Therapy. *J Pain Symptom Management* 1997;14:S14. **Kamran S, Wright BD.** Complications of intrathecal drug delivery systems. *Neuromodulation* 2001;4:111.

N. Spinal cord stimulators (SCS)

The use of spinal cord stimulators (SCS) has become more common. Electrodes are implanted in the dorsal epidural space and connected to a pulse generator. Paresthesias are elicited for pain relief over the distribution of pain. In 1967, the first "dorsal column" stimulator was developed. It slowly gained popularity over the next few decades. In the 1980's, the first programmable electrode system was introduced in the U.S. In 1982, SCS that is completely implantable under the skin was used for the first time. There have been well over 150,000 implantations of neurostimulation systems so far.

The exact *mechanism of action* for pain control is not known. However, there are at least five theories that may explain the mechanism: 1) gate control theory with segmental, antidromic activation of A-beta efferents; 2) neurotransmission block via the spinothalamic tract; 3) supraspinal pain inhibition; 4) activation of central inhibitory mechanisms which affect the sympathetic efferent neurons; or 5) activation of "putative" neurotransmitters or neuromodulators. It's not likely that a lone model completely explains its mechanism of action by itself; rather, multiple mechanisms are probably operating sequentially or simultaneously (Oakley and Prager, 2002).

Indications and patient selection - Indications include post-laminectomy syndrome (failed back surgery syndrome), radiculopathies, complex regional pain syndrome, postamputation pain, postherpetic neuralgia, peripheral neuropathy, spinal cord injury, dysesthesias, multiple sclerosis, angina pectoris, peripheral vascular disease, Raynaud's disease, and pelvic pain.

Ideal candidates should be emotionally stable (except for depression on the Minnesota Multiphasic Personality Inventory), demonstrate acceptable medication usage and cooperation with the rehabilitation program. The literature suggests that an increased time interval from the onset of pain to SCS implantation decreases the likelihood of a positive response (Kumar, 2006). Other clinical trials and reports have compared spinal cord stimulation with re-operation, with favorable results for spinal cord stimulation (North, 2005; Taylor, 2005). While there is evidence favoring efficacy of spinal cord stimulators for post-laminectomy syndrome and complex regional pain syndrome, its efficacy in other types of chronic pain remain debatable (Mailis-Gagnon, 2004). Spinal cord stimulation has been shown to improve pain intensity, mood and quality of life (Burchiel, 1996).

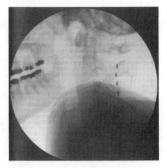

Figure 15n Spinal cord stimulator in the cervical spine.

An SCS "trial" is often performed with temporary leads to determine if the patient would benefit from a permanent implantation. A typical SCS trial involves patient going home after the placement of temporary SCS leads. The patient tries to go about his or her daily activity with the temporary SCS leads. If there is at least 50% improvement in pain and function during the trial period, a permanent implantation is considered.

Contraindications include previous failure of a SCS trial, implantable cardiac pacemaker or defibrillator, diathermy, infection, coagulopathy, poor patient compliance or inability to operate the system, and systemic infection. Safety has not been established in pregnant or pediatric patients.

Equipment - Leads can be implanted percutaneously or with laminotomy. The distribution of paresthesias is determined by the position of the stimulating anodes and cathodes. Pulse generator implanted with the leads is powered by a battery, which can last from 3–5 years. Rechargeable models are also available with battery life guaranteed for at least 5 years, and sometimes longer. An external patient programmer via a radiofrequency signal programs the pulse generator. Patients themselves can change stimulus amplitude, pulse width and rate using a hand-held programmer.

Adverse events include jolting or shocking, hematoma, epidural hemorrhage, seroma, CSF leakage, infection, erosion, allergic response, hardware malfunction or migration, pain at implant site, loss of pain relief, chest wall stimulation, spinal cord injury, and associated surgical risks.

Refs: Oakley JC, Prager JP. Spinal cord stimulation: mechanisms of action. *Spine* 2002;27:2574; **Mailis-Gagnon A, et al.** Spinal cord stimulation for chronic pain. *Cochrane Database Syst Rev* 2004;3:CD003783; **Kumar K, et al.** Spinal cord stimulation in treatment of chronic benign pain: challenges in treatment planning and present status, a 22-year experience. *Neurosurg* 2006;58:481; **North RB, et al.** Spinal cord stimulation versus repeated lumbosacral spine surgery for chronic pain: a randomized, controlled trial. *Neurosurgery* 2005;56(1):98; **Burchiel KJ, et al.** Prospective, multicenter study of spinal cord stimulation for relief of chronic back and extremity pain. *Spine* 1996;21:2786; **Taylor RS, et al.** Spinal cord stimulation for chronic back and leg pain and failed back surgery syndrome: a systematic review and analysis of prognostic factors. *Spine.* 2005;30:152. **Figure credit: 15n.** Radiograph courtesy of **Ballantyne JC.** *The MGH Handbook of Pain Management*, 3rd ed. Philadelphia, LWW, 2006, with permission.

Ch.16: COMPLEMENTARY AND ALTERNATIVE MEDICINE (CAM)

Complementary and alternative medicine (CAM) is increasingly being utilized as part of comprehensive treatment of pain. The NIH National Center for Complementary and Alternative Medicine (NCCAM) classifies CAM therapies into five categories (examples of each are included):

1) *Alternative Medical Systems* - based on complete systems of theory and practice, including Ayurvedic medicine (native to India); homeopathy (developed by a German physician, Samuel Hahnemann); and acupuncture (based on maintaining balanced "chi" or energy in the body).

2) *Mind-body interventions* - the goal is to enhance the mind's ability to affect bodily functions. Examples include:

Hypnotherapy - successful pain relief in cases of chronic back pain and for headaches following brain injury has been anecdotally reported; published controlled studies, however, have not used equally credible placebos or minimally effective pain treatment, so conclusions about the effectiveness of hypnotic therapy as an analgesic over and above its effects on patient expectancy are difficult to make (Jensen, 2006).

Meditation - involves "quieting the mind" while focusing on a single stimulus such as breathing or a mantra. A randomized, controlled trial of breath therapy vs. extensive PT demonstrated improved VAS scores, function, and SF-36 scores in both groups, with trends favoring breath therapy at 6–8 wks and favoring PT at 6 months (Mehling, 2005).

A pilot study demonstrated that a 10 wk group outpatient program for patients with fibromyalgia lowered many pain measures, SCL-90-R, Fibromyalgia Impact Questionnaire, and Fibromyalgia Attitude Index scores vs. pre-intervention levels in all patients, with 51% showing moderate to marked improvement (Kaplan, 1993).

Movement therapies - include yoga, Tai chi and dance. Goals include improving kinesthetic ability, posture, range of motion and providing an emotional outlet, while reducing pain.

There are many schools of yoga, which may differ in their emphasis of various aspects of yoga: body alignment, breath/movement coordination, or holding postures. A randomized, controlled trial of yoga (12 wk program), therapeutic exercise (12 wks), and a self-help book in patients with chronic low back pain showed improvement in the yoga group in back-related function above the exercise and book groups at 12 wks, and above the book group at 26 wks (Sherman, 2005).

Tai chi, often translated as "supreme ultimate force," is typically practiced as a meditative exercise consisting of soft, graceful movements. A Cochrane review of Tai chi for rheumatoid arthritis (RA) concluded that Tai chi does not exacerbate RA symptoms, while ROM in the lower limbs, especially ankles, was improved. Effects on pain were not examined by the studies in the literature reviewed (Han, 2004). A single-blind, randomized study involving 66 subjects reported potential usefulness of tai chi for fibromyalgia (Wang, 2010).

Biofeedback - patients learn to control muscle tension via auditory or visual feedback they receive from a biofeedback device that measures muscle activity via surface EMG electrodes. There are no recent high-grade studies in pain medicine. Trials in the 1980s showed mixed results in terms of long-term efficacy (Bush, 1985; Flor, 1986).

3) *Biologically based therapies* - examples include: herbals and dietary supplements. High-grade studies for some of the more widely used therapies have

recently been completed or are now underway. Most therapies, however, have only anecdotal support. In the U.S., these substances are not subject to the same FDA regulations as conventional pharmaceuticals.

A Cochrane review found encouraging results in medium to high quality trials supporting the efficacy of *Harpagophytum procumbens* (**Devil's claw**), *Salix alba* (**white willow**), and *Capsicum frutescens* (**cayenne pepper**) treatments over placebo for low back pain (Gagnier, 2006). Feverfew, a remedy described in folklore to be helpful for headaches and arthritis, contains parthenolide as its main active ingredient, an inhibitor of prostaglandins and leukotrienes. A small double-blinded trial, however, did not demonstrate any benefit of feverfew over placebo for rheumatoid arthritis pain (Pattrick, 1989). A Cochrane review revealed no clear evidence of benefit of feverfew in preventing migraine (Pittler, 2004).

The multicenter, randomized, double-blinded, placebo and celecoxib-controlled **Glucosamine/chondroitin** Arthritis Intervention Trial (GAIT) did not demonstrate efficacy of either agent alone over placebo, but (on exploratory analyses) demonstrated some potential benefit for the combination of the two in subgroups with moderate to severe knee pain (Clegg, 2006).

4) *Manipulative and body-based methods* - the quality of trials for massage in mechanical neck pain and LBP is low (Haraldsson, 2006; Furlan, 2010). There is some evidence that massage may be beneficial for patients with subacute and chronic LBP, especially when combined with exercises and education. Acupressure massage may be more effective than classic (Swedish) massage, but confirmation is needed. Functional benefits, however, have not been demonstrated to date, and cost-effectiveness is unclear (Furlan, 2010).

Manipulation - although based on different philosophies, osteopaths, chiropractors, and physical therapists use manipulation to treat pain. It is a passive mechanical treatment applied to a specific vertebral region with the goal of restoring lost vertebral motion.

Manipulation under anesthesia (MUA) - as stated in the Guidelines for Chiropractic Quality Assurance and Practice Parameters ("Mercy Document"), MUA is an "equivocal" therapy meaning that the benefits of the procedure are not clearly established. Many chiropractors, however, have not agreed with the overall findings and recommendations of the Mercy Document. There is scattered support in the literature in the form of non-high-grade evidence, such as case reports and case series. There have also been, however, reports of iatrogenic intraarticular damage due to MUA (Loew, 2005). Individual cases must be reviewed on an ad hoc basis to determine whether the potential benefits from a functional and/or quality of life standpoint outweigh the potential risks of MUA, including the anesthesia risks.

Myofascial release involves palpation to locate "restricted" areas of connective tissue, followed by gentle stretch until a softening or release is felt. Although there are intuitively many benefits to myofascial release (not unlike massage therapy) such as temporary pain and stress relief, there is as yet no evidence in the medical literature demonstrating long-term sustained benefits with respect to function, mobility or pain relief.

Craniosacral therapy involves the palpation of "craniosacral rhythms" (purported externally appreciable CNS/ CSF rhythms, not related to the cardiovascular rhythm) which proponents believe can be adjusted by gentle manipulation (e.g., the cranial sutures) to treat headaches, spinal pains and other ailments. While the brain does pulsate due to blood flow, interrater reliability in the palpatory measurement of alleged craniosacral rhythms has not been demonstrated to date.

5) *Energy therapies* - many practices stem from Anton Mesmer's theory (18th century) that "energy fields," which can extend beyond the body, can be manipulated to influence health.

Therapeutic touch - proponents typically claim that energy can be transferred from practitioner to patient through touch (or from proximity in the non-contact version). Reiki is a Japanese term meaning "universal life energy." Practitioners believe they can redirect and balance the energy of patients through the placement of hands in various positions on or near the patient's body. Advanced practitioners of reiki claim to have healing powers over remote distances.

Static magnetic therapy - is popular for many types of pain. Some pilot studies have suggested efficacy while others have not. Rigorous clinical trials are complicated, however, by the lack of a credible placebo (i.e., subjects can easily detect placebo magnets). A popular misconception that the iron in hemoglobin can affected by magnetic fields (which might support the contention that circulation can be stimulated by magnetic therapy) is untrue as the iron in blood is not ferromagnetic.

Ref: Jensen M, Patterson DR. Hypnotic treatment of chronic pain. *J Behav Med* 2006;29:95; **Mehling WE, et al.** Randomized, controlled trial of breath therapy for patients with chronic LBP. *Altern Ther Health Med* 2005;11:44; **Kaplan KH, et al.** The impact of a meditation-based stress reduction program on fibromyalgia. *Gen Hosp Psychiatry* 1993;15:284; **Sherman KJ, et al.** Comparing yoga, exercise, and a self-care book for chronic LBP: a randomized, controlled trial. *Ann Intern Med* 2005;143:849; **Han A, et al.** Tai chi for treating RA. *Cochrane Database Syst Rev* 2004;(3):CD004849; **Wang C, et al.** A randomized trial of tai chi for fibromyalgia. *NEJM* 2010;363:743; **Bush C, et al.** A controlled evaluation of paraspinal EMG biofeedback in the treatment of chronic LBP. *Health Psychol* 1985;4:307; **Flor H, et al.** Long-term efficacy of EMG biofeedback for chronic rheumatic back pain. *Pain* 1986;27:195; **Clogg DO, et al.** Glucosamine, chondroitin, and the two in combination for painful knee arthritis. *NEJM* 2006;354:795; **Gagnier JJ, et al.** Herbal medicine for LBP. *Cochrane Database Syst Rev* 2006;(2):CD004504; **Pattrick M, et al.** Feverfew in RA: a double-blind, placebo controlled study. *Ann Rheum Dis* 1986;48:547; **Pittler MH, et al.** Feverfew for preventing migraine. *Cochrane Database Syst Rev* 2004;(1):CD002286; **Haraldsson BG, et al.** Massage for mechanical neck disorders. *Cochrane Database Syst Rev* 2006;(3):CD004871; **Furlan AD, et al.** Massage for LBP: an updated systematic review within the framework of the Cochrane Back Review Group. *Spine* 2009;34:1669; **Haldeman S, et al.** Guidelines for Chiropractic Quality Assurance and Practice Parameters: Proceedings of the Mercy Center Consensus Conference. 1993, Aspen Publishers; **Loew M, et al.** Intraarticular lesions in primary frozen shoulder after manipulation under general anesthesia. *J Shoulder Elbow Surg* 2005;14:16.

ACUPUNCTURE

According to traditional Chinese medicine (TCM), "chi," a vital energy force, flows through 12 "meridians" (each corresponding to an organ) throughout the body (see figure, right). Disturbances of this flow lead to pain and disease. Acupuncture points along the meridians can be stimulated to dissipate or tonify (restore) chi. "De Chi" is a deep aching, tingling sensation felt by the patient upon needling the acupuncture points. De Chi is believed to be necessary for therapeutic effect. Adverse effects are usually mild and include bruising, bleeding, and a transient vasovagal response.

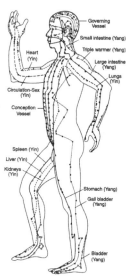

Scientific basis - scientific data has suggested that acupuncture needling results in multiple physiological effects, including:
- the stimulation of GABA receptors in the CNS (blocking messages from peripheral nociceptors) and activating of the raphe descending system;
- the production of endorphins in the CNS;
- the production of immunomodulatory factors (i.e., the acupuncture needle acts as a foreign body to increase ACTH levels which, in turn, stimulates production of corticosteroids);
- affecting the gene expression of neurohormones;
- modulation of the hypothalamic-limbic systems and subcortical structures (demonstrated on functional MRI).

Clinical studies - have generally been limited by suboptimal designs, especially the lack of a good placebo control (until recently). The results of higher quality trials have been equivocal. Major trials and reviews include:
- the NIH consensus panel, 1997/1998: hundreds of studies were reviewed, with mostly equivocal findings due to design issues; promising results were noted in chemotherapy-induced nausea, dental pain, nausea of pregnancy, and postoperative nausea. Potentially useful indications included: addiction, asthma, carpal tunnel syndrome, epicondylitis, fibromyalgia, headache, low back pain, stroke, and menstrual cramps;
- a large randomized controlled trial (RCT) demonstrated significant effectiveness of acupuncture as an adjunctive therapy in osteoarthritis of the knee (Berman, 2004);
- a prospective, partially-blinded RCT showed significant improvement of pain, fatigue, and anxiety symptoms in patients with fibromyalgia (Martin, 2006);
- a RCT demonstrated addition of acupuncture (both TCM and sham acupuncture groups) resulted in better control of pain and improved function compared to conventional treatment for knee arthritis alone; however, no difference between the TCM acupuncture and sham acupuncture groups was noted, suggesting benefits could be due to the placebo effect or the physiological effect of needling (Scharf, 2006);

• A meta-analysis (Manheimer, 2007) reported that sham-controlled trials show clinically irrelevant short-term benefits of acupuncture for treating knee osteoarthritis. Waiting list–controlled trials suggest clinically relevant benefits, some of which may be due to placebo or expectation effects.

Conclusions and the future - Traditionally, the clinical literature has suffered from poor design, but more recently, well-designed studies with proper controls have been proliferating and a scientific basis for acupuncture is emerging. Nevertheless, while needling appears to have beneficial clinical effects, it is still unclear whether acupuncture confers benefits beyond the placebo effect and whether the strict application of TCM principles is necessary for the effect. Nascent cost-effectiveness literature, however, suggests that acupuncture may nevertheless play an increasing role within Western medicine, particularly given the high costs and uncertain efficacies of many conventional and alternative therapies.

Ref: Stux G, et al. Scientific basis of acupuncture: acupuncture textbook and atlas. New York, Springer Verlag, 1987; **NIH Consensus Conference:** Acupuncture. *JAMA* 1998;280:1518; **Berman BM et al.** Effectiveness of acupuncture as adjunctive therapy in OA of the knee: a RCT. *Ann Intern Med* 2004;141:901; **Martin DP.** Improvement in fibromyalgia symptoms with acupuncture: results of a RCT. *Mayo Clin Proc* 2006;81:749; **Scharf HP, et al**. Acupuncture and knee OA: a 3-armed randomized trial. *Ann Intern Med* 2006;145:12; **Manheimer E, et al.** Meta-analysis: Acupuncture for Osteoarthritis of the Knee. *Ann Int Med* 2007;146:868. **Figure credit:** Courtesy of **Loeser JD, et al.**, eds. *Bonica's Management of Pain*, 3rd ed. Philadelphia, LWW, 2001, with permission.

Part Three
Specific Syndromes and Miscellaneous

Ch.17: HEADACHE

The U.S. prevalence of headache (HA) is 78% for females and 68% for males (Taylor, 1985). 40% of Americans have severe, debilitating HA at least once in life (Ballantyne, 2002). The vast majority of patients will suffer from recurrent headaches.

Pain-sensitive structures include extracranial structures, meningeal arteries, 5th, 9th, 10th cranial nerves, venous sinuses, meninge, dura, and upper 3 cervical nerves. Pain-insensitive structures include the brain parenchyma, pia, and arachnoid. A primary headache is a headache with no clear underlying structural, infectious or systemic abnormality.

Migraine headache
Migraines are syndromes consisting of paroxysmal headaches associated with other signs and symptoms, typically lasting anywhere between 4 and 72 hours. There are 5 stages to the migraine: prodrome, aura, pain/headache, resolution, and postdrome. Common triggers include hormonal changes (e.g., menstrual cycle), foods (e.g., chocolate), weather changes, skipped meals, and stress. There is a 3:1 female:male ratio.

Pathophysiological theories include: 1) the vasogenic theory, where intracranial vasoconstriction is responsible for aura, with headache resulting from rebound dilation and vaso-active polypeptides; and 2) the neurogenic theory, where a lower cerebral threshold with acute cortical spreading depression (neuronal depolarization), believed to originate in the occipital lobe and spreading rostrally, results in an aura and subsequent vascular headache.

Some migraine subtypes include:
1) migraine without aura (formerly, common migraine)
2) migraine with aura (classic migraine)
3) basilar migraine
4) migraine with prolonged aura
5) familial hemiplegic migraine
6) migraine without headache
7) status migrainosus (lasting for >72 hrs)

Migraine without aura (formerly, common migraine) is defined as follows (International Headache Society criteria):
   A. At least 5 attacks fulfilling criteria B-D
   B. Headache attacks lasting 4–72 hrs
   C. Headache has at least two of the following:
      1. unilateral
      2. pulsating
      3. moderate or severe pain
      4. aggravated by routine physical activity
   D. During headache at least one of the following:
      1. nausea and/or vomiting
      2. photophobia and phonophobia
   E. Not attributed to another disorder

Migraine with aura (formerly, classic migraine) is defined as follows (International Headache Society criteria):
   A. At least 2 attacks fulfilling criteria B-D
   B. Aura consisting of at least one of the following, but with no motor weakness:
      1. fully reversible visual symptoms
      2. fully reversible sensory symptoms
      3. fully reversible dysphasic speech disturbance

C. At least two of the following:
  1. homonymous visual symptoms and/or unilateral sensory symptoms
  2. one or more aura symptoms develop over ≥ 5 min
  3. each symptom lasts ≥ 5 min and ≤ 60 min
D. Headache fulfilling criteria B-D for migraine without aura begins during the aura or follows aura within 60 min
E. Not attributed to another disorder

Treatment for migraines includes abortive treatment, treatment of associated symptoms, and preventive treatment.

Abortive treatments for mild to moderate attacks include NSAIDs, acetaminophen, and caffeine.

For severe attacks, options include the selective serotonin agonists (e.g., sumatriptan 20 mg intranasally, 6 mg SC, or 25–50 mg oral) and nonspecific serotonin agonists (ergotamine or nasal/IM dihydroergotamine [DHE-45]). Caution must be taken with concomitant PVD or CAD because of the vasoconstrictive nature of serotonin agonists. Butalbital (barbituate + caffeine + acetaminophen/ASA) should be used sparingly due to the potential for dependence. For the same reason, opioids should be avoided.

Treatment of associated symptoms includes metoclopramide (Reglan) and promethazine (Phenergan).

Preventive treatments include beta blockers (atenolol 10–30 mg bid, propanolol 10–80 mg tid), tricyclic antidepressants, and clonidine.

Treatment for status migrainosus may require inpatient admission, particularly due to risk of stroke. Treatment consists of IV DHE-45 10 mg with or without IV metoclopramide 10 mg. Dopamine antagonists, opioids, SC sumatriptan, and supportive IV fluids are other options. A sphenopalatine block can also be considered.

Tension-type headache

Tension headaches are the most common headache disorder. There are episodic or chronic forms. The etiology is unclear, although it is generally felt to originate in the muscles. The diagnosis requires 10 headaches with the following features:
  1) Headache 30 minutes to 7 days
  2) At least 2 of the following
    a. Pressing/tightening quality (Non-pulsatile)
    b. Mild to moderate (not prohibiting normal activities)
    c. Bilateral
    d. Not aggravated by activity
  3) Both of the following
    a. no nausea of vomiting
    b. no more than one of photophobia or phonophobia
  4) Not attributed to another disorder

Treatment consists of rest, physical modalities, minor analgesics, muscle relaxants (baclofen), and tricyclic antidepressants.

Cluster headache

Cluster headaches are much less common, although it is six times more common in men than women. Attacks occur in clusters lasting weeks or months, separated by remissions that last for months or years. Triggers include alcohol, histamine, nitroglycerin. In contrast to migraine, patient classically paces the room. Associated with lacrimation, nasal drainage, papillary changes, and conjunctival injection. The diagnosis requires at least 5 attacks with the following criteria:
  1) Severe unilateral orbital or supra-orbital and/or temporal pain lasting 15–180 minutes.

2) At least one of the following on the ipsilateral side: a. conjunctival injection; b. nasal congestion/rhinorrhea; c. eyelid edema; d. forehead and facial sweating; e. miosis and/or ptosis; f. restless or agitation.
3) At least one attack every other day up to 8 attacks/day.
4) There is no other identifiable cause.

Treatment consists of 100% oxygen administered with face-mask, intranasal lidocaine/sphenopalatine block, intranasal lidocaine 4% (drops or spray), serotonin agonist (triptan or DHE), IV glucocorticoids. Steroids, verapamil, and lithium have been used for prevention during cluster period.

Chronic daily headache

Evolves from migraine or tension-type headaches. It is often related to drug overuse. Treatment includes medication simplification and detoxification.

Other types of primary headache include cervicogenic; occipital neuralgia; chronic paroxysmal hemicrania (responsive to indomethacin); paroxysmal hemicrania, hemicrania continua; idiopathic stabbing headache; benign exertional headache; cold-induced headache (the ice-cream headache); and coital headache.

Secondary headache include vasculogenic (subarachnoid or the "worst headache of [my] life", subdural, epidural hemorrhage, AV malformation, and CVA-related headaches), neoplastic, infectious, inflammatory, hypertensive, glaucoma, drug withdrawl, elevated ICP, and post-traumatic (post-concussive) headaches.

Key points regarding headache management:

First, identify which of the three groups patient's headache belongs to:
   1. 1st time severe headache (high index of suspicion for intracranial process)
   2. History of chronic headache but recent change in frequency, character, or intensity
   3. Chronic paroxysmal headache

Determine if it is a primary vs. secondary headache with history and neurologic exam. Use imaging as needed. It's imperative not to miss a subarachnoid hemorrhage's sentinel headache. Important questions include:
   a. First headache like this?
   b. Did this begin suddenly?
   c. Recent infection/trauma?
   d. Does this occur with exertion?

If the patient is a woman, ask if they may be pregnant prior to initiating treatment. Avoid over-medication. Taper off if headache-free for a few months. Optimize non-pharmacologic management: Avoidance of triggers, environmental modification (quiet, dark room during migraine), biofeedback, and psychological management are important part of the management.

Ref: Taylor H, Curran NM. *The Nuprin Pain Report.* NY, Louis Harris & Associates, 1985; **Ballantyne JC.** *The MGH Handbook of Pain Management,* 2nd ed. p. 389–410, 2002; **Loeser JD, et al., eds.** Bonica's Management of Pain, 3rd ed. Philadelphia, LWW, 2001:867–894; **Headache Classification Committee of the International Headache Society.** The International Classification of Headache Disorders: 2nd ed. *Cephalalgia* 2004;24(S1):9.

Ch.18: NEUROPATHIC PAIN

Neuropathic pain is a complex disorder initiated by a primary lesion or dysfunction in the nervous system (Merskey, 1994). Common causes include diabetes, alcohol, herpes zoster infection, HIV-related neuropathies, toxins, malignancy-related pain, genetic disorders, and immune mediated disorders. It develops as a consequence of changes in the affected neurons and results in a chronically sustained, spontaneously-occuring pain. In contrast to nociceptive pain which has a crucial, protective role by warning the body of impending or active tissue damage, neuropathic pain is not thought to have a useful biological function.

Neuropathic and nociceptive pain often coexist. It is necessary to distinguish the two entities when formulating a rational and effective treatment plan.

Mechanisms for nerve injury and neuropathic pain are multifactorial, complex and evolve over time. Peripheral and central sensitizations are two proposed models to explain the development of neuropathic pain. Reorganizational changes can occur at the level of the dorsal horn following a peripheral nerve injury. For example, low-threshold mechanoreceptors have been shown to sprout from deep laminae and synapse in laminae I and II of the dorsal horn after peripheral nerve injury.

Peripheral sensitization is a phenomenon involving lowering of nociceptor depolarization threshold and ectopic discharges that occur after nerve injury. It may lead to chronic neuropathic pain. The proposed mechanism is a release of inflammatory mediators that occur after nerve injury. Namely, neuropeptides (substance P) from primary afferent nociceptors and prostaglandins (PGE2) from sympathetic postganglionic neurons are thought to be involved. These substances activate nearby receptors and trigger a process of spreading activation. This leads to accumulation and altered expression of sodium channels in the axon membranes and dorsal root ganglia. Consequently, this results in lowering of nociceptor depolarization threshold and in ectopic discharges.

Central sensitization refers to a phenomenon involving sensitization of nociceptors in the dorsal horn of the spinal cord following injury to the peripheral tissues. Proposed mechanism involves the release of tachykinins (substance P, neurokinin A) from peripheral nociceptors after peripheral nerve injury, triggering release of calcium and facilitating upregulation of NMDA receptors in the dorsal horn cells. This leads to the release of excitatory neurotransmitters (e.g., glutamate) from primary afferents, leading to additional influx of calcium into the cells. The intracellular calcium influx triggers a cascade of enzymatic and genetic activity with long-term consequences, including (1) lowering of threshold of spinal horn neurons; (2) increase in magnitude and duration of the responses to stimuli; (3) "wind-up" phenomenon or prolonged discharge of dorsal horn cells secondary to repetitive noxious stimulation of unmyelinated C-fibers; and (4) expansion in the size of the receptive field.

Treatments

Tricyclic antidepressants (TCAs) are strong Na channel modulators and are among the most effective treatments for neuropathic pain. They can have modulatory effects on descending inhibitory pathways. TCAs, from the least to most side effects, include: desipramine, nortriptyline, imipramine, doxepin, and amitriptyline.

Anticonvulsants are widely used. Their antineuralgic effect is through their effect on sodium channels, suppressing spontaneous ectopic discharges.

• *Gabapentin* has a favorable side-effect profile. Its exact mechanism of action is unknown but it is known to bind to α2δ subunit of the voltage-dependent calcium channel in the neurons. It may act synergetistically with opioids (Gilron, 2005). It is FDA approved for postherpetic neuralgia and is also used off-label in the treatment of various other neuropathic pain conditions. Pregabalin, which followed gabapentin, is FDA approved for pain associated with diabetic neuropathy and fibromyalgia.

- *Topiramate* works via GABA receptors to limit sustained repetitive discharges.
- *Carbamazepine* is structurally related to the TCAs. It reduces high-frequency repetitive firing of Na channel action, inhibiting ectopic discharges. FDA approved for trigeminal neuralgia.
- *Oxcarbazepine* is a keto-analog of carbamazepine.
- *Lamotrigine* is structurally unrelated to other anticonvulsants. It stabilizes slow inactivated conformation of Na channels and inhibits repetitive firing of action potentials under conditions of sustained neuronal depolarization. It is the drug of choice for HIV-associated neuropathic pain.

Traditional analgesics (NSAIDs) are relatively ineffective in the treatment of neuropathic pain. Opioids are effective in some neuropathic pains. Tramadol is a weak μ-agonist that also inhibits serotonin/norepinephrine reuptake. The lidocaine transdermal patch (Lidoderm) is FDA approved for postherpetic neuralgia. Capsaicin releases substance P from peripheral and central C-fiber terminals, depleting substance P over time. IV lidocaine and oral mexiletine reduce neuropathic pain.

Some choices for various neuropathic pains include:
- trigeminal neuralgia: carbamazepine, lamotrigine, oxcarbazepine
- central post-stroke pain: lamotrigine
- postherpetic neuralgia: gabapentin, pregabalin
- diabetic neuropathy: carbamazepine, phenytoin, gabapentin, lamotrigine, pregabalin

Ref: **Merskey H, Bogduk N eds.** Classification of Chronic Pain, 2nd ed. Seattle, IASP Press, 1994; **Rowbotham MC, et al.** Gabapentin for the treatment of postherpetic neuralgia: a randomized controlled trial. *JAMA* 1998;280:1837; **Sindrup SH, Jensen TS.** Efficacy of pharmacological treatments of neuropathic pain: update and effect related to mechanism of drug action. *Pain* 1999;83:389; **Gilron I, et al.** Morphine, Gabapentin, or Their Combination for Neuropathic Pain. *NEJM* 2005;352:1324.

Ch.19: FIBROMYALGIA AND MYOFASCIAL PAIN

FIBROMYALGIA is a chronic pain disorder characterized by widespread musculoskeletal aches, pain and stiffness, soft tissue tenderness, general fatigue and sleep disturbances. The etiology of fibromyalgia is unclear. It is estimated that approximately 3–6% of the U.S. population has fibromyalgia. While about 80% of those diagnosed are women, fibromyalgia may be seen with any gender, age, or ethnicity.

The most common sites of pain include the neck, back, shoulders, pelvic girdle and hands, but any body part can be involved. The pain is severe, widespread and chronic. Often, fibromyalgia pain has been described as deep muscular aching, throbbing, twitching, stabbing, and shooting, and it often consumes the patient's life. Neurological complaints such as numbness, tingling, and burning often coexist and add to the discomfort of the patient.

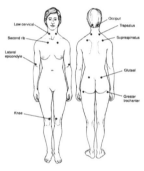

Genetics play a role in fibromyalgia, with strong patterns of familial aggregation. Mode of inheritance is unknown but likely polygenic. Polymorphisms of genes in the serotonergic, dopaminergic, and catecholaminergic systems may play a role in etiology (Smith, 2010).

Fibromyalgia adversely impacts function and activities of daily living. Chronic pain appears to have major impact on mental health and social functioning (Carmona, 2001).

Fibromyalgia affects sleep quality. Analysis of EEG indicates that the patients with fibromyalgia take longer to fall alseep, have frequent arousals, show extended stage 1 sleep, and demonstrate little slow wave sleep, indicative of vigilant arousal state during sleep (Bigatti, 2008).

Figure 19 According to the American College of Rheumatology criteria, pain in 11 or more of the above 18 predetermined tender points are seen in fibromyalgia (Wolfe, 1990).

Diagnosis: Diagnosis of fibromyalgia is based on history and clinical findings of tender points on palpation as per the American College of Rheumatology criteria. The ACR criteria stipulate that pain be present for at least 3 months, be present on both sides of the body, and exist above as well as below the waist. Patients should be tender at a minimum of 11 out of 18 designated tender points (all bilateral - suboccipital muscle insertion into the occiput, anterior aspect of interspace between transverse processes of C5–C7, midpoint of upper border of trapezius, medial border of scapula, 2nd rib at upper surface of costochondral junction, 2 cm distal to lateral epicondyle, upper outer quadrant of buttocks, greater trochanter, and medial knee fat pad). Fibromyalgia is a diagnosis of exclusion, although it should be noted that coexistence with another identifiable disease is possible.

Treatment: The mainstay consist of the three A's: analgesia, antidepressants, and aerobic exercise. Patient needs to recognize the need for lifestyle adaptation. Other therapies that may be helpful include physical therapy, therapeutic massage, myofascial release therapy, aquatic therapy, application of heat or cold, acupressure, acupuncture, yoga, relaxation exercises, breathing techniques, aromatherapy, cognitive therapy, biofeedback, herbs, nutritional supplements, and osteopathic or chiropractic manipulations as well as tai chi. Ideally, the practitioner should establish a multifaceted and individualized approach that works for the patient.

Pain management: OTC medications such as acetaminophen or ibuprofen may be helpful in relieving pain. Also available are newer analgesics (e.g., tramadol) or low doses of antidepressants (e.g., tricyclic antidepressants, serotonin reuptake inhibitors). If the patient is experiencing depression, higher levels of these or other medications may need to be prescribed. Newer agents such as pregabalin, duloxetine and milnacipran have been FDA-approved for treatments of fibromyalgia.

Sleep hygiene: Sleep disturbance has been proposed as a predictor of pain and depression in patients with fibromyalgia (Bigatti, 2008). Good sleep hygiene is therefore important in the management of fibromyalgia. Regular sleep schedule should be encouraged. Sleep environment should be free from distractions. Stimulants and alcohol should be avoided before bedtime.

Psychological support: Strategies to cope with chronic conditions such as fibromyalgia are crucial. Support system through family, friends and places of worship are often helpful and can serve as important sources of emotional support. Local and national chapters with support groups for fibromyalgia exist.

There is evidence that psychological interventions are helpful in management of fibromyalgia. Cognitive behavioral therapies have been shown to improve coping with pain and reduce depressive symptoms (Bernardy, 2010).

Prognosis: For patients who adhere to comprehensive and multidisciplinary approach, treating their fibromyalgia symptoms can be effectively accomplished. The symptoms of fibromyalgia can vary in severity and often wax and wane, but with many patients have learned to cope with and function despite limitations caused imposed fibromyalgia.

Ref: Wolfe F, et al. The American College of Rheumatology 1990 Criteria for the Classification of Fibromyalgia. Report of the Multicenter Criteria Committee. *Arthritis Rheum* 1990;33:160; **Smith HS, Barkin RL.** Fibromyalgia syndrome: a discussion of the syndrome and pharmacotherapy. *Am J Ther* 2010;17:418; **Carmona L, et al.** The burden of musculoskeletal disease in the general population of Spain: results from a national survey. *Ann Rheum Dis* 2001;60:1040; **Bigatti SM, et al.** Sleep disturbance in fibromyalgia syndrome: relationship to pain and depression. *Arth & Rheum* 2008;59:961; **Bernardy K, et al.** Efficacy of cognitive-behavioral therapies in fibromyalgia syndrome - a systemic review and metaanalysis of randomized controlled trials. *J Rheum* 2010;37:1991. *Figure from LWW*

MYOFASCIAL PAIN SYNDROME is a chronic pain syndrome manifested by dysfunction of the muscle or connective tissue. It is usually limited to a specific region of the body, as opposed to affecting the body diffusely as may be seen in fibromyalgia. Biopsies have demonstrated no inflammation or EMG findings which led to the demise of the older terms such as fibromyositis. Myofascial pain is invariably associated with trigger points, which are characterized by (1) exquisite focal tenderness, (2) palpable taut bands, (3) local twitch response, and (4) reproduction of characteristic referred pain patterns as described by seminal works of Travell and Simons.

Criteria for myofascial pain syndrome:

A. Major criteria (active trigger points)
   1. Complaint of pain in a given region
   2. Taut band in muscle

   3. Marked local tenderness in muscle
   4. Referred pain, paresthesia or altered sensation at a site distant from the
      muscle point which "triggers" it
   5. Reproduction of the patient's pain on palpation of the trigger point

B. Minor criteria
   6. Restricted range of muscle lengthening with possible resultant loss of range
      of motion (minor) about a joint
   7. Weakness
   8. Autonomic dysfunction: piloerection or skin temperature changes

Condition 1–5 in A and at least one other in 6–8 must be present for diagnosis
(Simons, 1990).

Treatment options include 1. spray and stretch; 2. trigger point injections (22 to
25 gauge 1.5 to 3 inch needle) using a dry needling technique, or with saline or
local anesthetic infiltration. Injection should be followed by relative rest of the
injected muscle and 3 days of PT to include stretching and regular 20 min local
hot pack treatments; 3. botulinum toxin injections may be of help in select cases.

Ref: Simons D. Muscular Pain Syndrome. In Fricton JR and Awad EA, eds. Myofascial Pain and Fibromyalgia. *Advances in Pain Research and Therapy* Vol 17. Raven Press, 1990.

Ch.20: COMPLEX REGIONAL PAIN SYNDROME (CRPS)

CRPS is a chronic pain disorder characterized by pain, swelling and trophic change in the skin overlying the affected area. CRPS may be seen following trauma, stroke, MI, musculoskeletal disorder, or malignancy, or it may be idiopathic.

There are two types: CRPS Type I and Type II as defined by International Association for the Study of Pain (IASP). Diagnostic criteria (described by Merskey, 1994) are as follows:

CRPS Type I (reflex sympathetic dystrophy or RSD): In CRPS I, an initiating noxious event or immobilization is often present. There is continuing pain, allodynia, or hyperalgesia with the pain being disproportionate to the inciting event. There is often evidence of edema, changes in skin blood flow, or abnormal sudomotor (sweat gland) activity in the painful region at some point in the disease progression. Generally, there is an absence of other conditions that would explain the degree of pain and dysfunction.

CRPS Type II (causalgia) has same criteria as CRPS Type I, except the pain occurs after a definable nerve injury. There are no specific laboratory tests to diagnose CRPS. EMG and nerve conduction studies are typically normal. Imaging studies may show asymmetric skin temperatures (difference >0.6° C) on thermography. X-rays may demonstrate trophic changes such as patchy demineralization. The triple-phase bone scan is considered the most sensitive and specific, especially in the early stages. Sudomotor function test (e.g., sweat test), laser doppler imaging, and a response to diagnostic sympathetic ganglion block are other tests, with the caveat that a diagnostic sympathetic block is not pathognomonic for CRPS, and not all CRPS may respond to sympathetic ganglion block (Singh, 2008).

CRPS may affect almost any body part, although it is most commonly seen in the extremities. In one series, 65% of CRPS I cases was preceded by trauma (mostly fracture), followed by operation (19%) and inflammatory process (2%). In 10% of cases, no precipitating event could be found (Veldman, 1993). Proposed mechanisms include changes in the peripheral and central somatosensory, autonomic, and motor processing, and a pathologic interaction of sympathetic and afferent systems (Portenoy, 2003).

There is limited epidemiological data, but the incidence of CRPS II following injury to peripheral nerve has been reported to be as high as 5%. The incidence of CRPS I is 1–2% after various fractures, and 2–5% after peripheral nerve injury (Singh, 2008).

Common complaints and physical findings include pain (90%), edema (typically abnormal vasodilation and warm extremity initially, then cold and pale skin in later stages), sensory dysfunction (allodynia, hyperalgesia), altered motor function (weakness, tremor, muscle spasm, dystonia), and psychological dysfunction. Stages have been described: 1) acute or hyperemic stage characterized by warm extremity; 2) dystrophic or ischemic stage characterized by vasomotor instability; 3) atrophic phase characterized by cold extremity with atrophic changes. Progression of CRPS in three well-defined stages, however, have not been consistently demonstrated (Portenoy, 2003).

Differential diagnosis includes: carpal tunnel syndrome, degenerative disc disease, myofascial pain, muscle strain/sprain, fibromyalgia, spasticity, thoracic outlet syndrome, traumatic brachial plexopathy, and ischemic monomelic neuropathy.

Treatment: Early recognition and treatment of CRPS is key, as the disease is invariably more difficult to treat in the later stages. Common treatment options include:

Medications, with variable results reported. Options include: opioids, tramadol, NSAIDs, acetaminophen, antidepressants, anticonvulsants (gabapentin, carbamazepine), benzodiazepines and muscle relaxants for muscle spasms, corticosteroids, alpha-adrenergic blockers (prazosin, phenoxybenzamine), clonidine, and lidocaine patch. Other options include: physical and occupational therapy for progressive weight bearing, desensitization, increasing strength and flexibility; *home exercise program, sympathetic blocks* (stellate ganglion block for upper extremity), *spinal cord stimulators, surgical or chemical sympathectomy.* There is less supportive data for regional intravenous techniques. Ketamine infusion has been proposed as a treatment (Schwartzman, 2009). Poor results were reported with amputation (Dielissen et al., 1995).

Ref: Merskey H, ed. Classification of Chronic Pain, 2nd ed. IASP Task Force on Taxonomy. IASP Press, 1994; **Portenoy R.** Neuropathic Pain. In Kanner R, ed: Pain Management Secrets, 2nd ed, Hanley & Belfus, 2003; **Singh M.** Complex Regional Pain Syndromes. http://emedicine.medscape.com/article/328054-overview, 2008; **Veldman PH, et al.** Signs and symptoms of reflex sympathetic dystrophy: prospective study of 829 patients. *Lancet* 1993;342:1012; **Schwartzman RJ, et al.** Outpatient intravenous ketamine for the treatment of complex regional pain syndrome: a double-blind placebo controlled study. *Pain* 2009;147:107; **Dielissen PW, et al.** Amputation for reflex sympathetic dystrophy. *J Bone Joint Surg Br* 1995;77:270.

Ch.21: CHRONIC NON-MALIGNANT PAIN AND SUBSTANCE ABUSE

The prevalence and societal costs of chronic nonmalignant pain (CNP) in the U.S. are high. A criteria for use of the term include: 1) pain of at least 3 months of duration; 2) a non-life-threatening or terminal condition; and 3) a lack of a brisk response to available treatments.

Assessment: Given the subjective nature of pain, monitoring of functional abilities, workplace activities, and social participation can be helpful in the overall assessment of patients with chronic pain. Assessment for mood disorders such as depression and anxiety is important given their high prevalence in CNP population. Suicide risk in those with CNP is high. If opioid analgesics are used, monthly prescriptions and frequent evaluations for treatment efficacy, tolerance (thought to be mediated by NMDA-receptor-related mechanisms), and side effects may be necessary.

Treatment: Therapy for those with CNP often requires analgesics. While the use of opioid analgesics is the treatment of choice in severe acute pain or in malignant pain, the use of opioids in CNP is controversial. Opioids allow for powerful analgesia without a ceiling effect, but chronic usage can be complicated by dependence and addiction.

The goal of treatment should be the elimination or reduction of pain to tolerable levels to maximize function. Encouraging and monitoring for follow through on goals is critical, as is the development of self-help and coping skills. Treating patients as addicts is inappropriate, as is the sudden withdrawal of opioids or sedative muscle relaxants. If the adverse effects of opioid therapy outweigh the benefits or if the therapy is not effective, dose reductions should be considered. As a guideline, dosages of medications can be reduced by 10% every 2–5 days, although the tapering schedule may be significantly slower for those with a more chronic history of medication use. Opioid withdrawal can present as a flu-like syndrome consisting of rhinorrhea, abdominal cramps, diarrhea, and piloerection.

Substance abuse costs the U.S. more than $484 billion per year, including health care expenditures, lost earnings, and costs associated with crime and accidents. Psychological stress is one of the most powerful triggers of substance abuse in susceptible individuals and of relapse in former addicts.

Addiction terminology - "History of substance abuse" is a vague term that can mean many different things. Use of the following addiction termionology, as defined by consensus from the American Academy of Pain Medicine, American Pain Society, and American Society of Addiction Medicine (Savage, 2003), is advocated:

Physical dependence - is a normal, physiologic state of adaptation to a drug. When physically dependent on a drug, a class-specific withdrawal syndrome can result from rapid dose reduction or abrupt cessation of the drug, decreasing blood levels of the drug, and/or administration of an antagonist. Symptoms during withdrawal can be prevented or treated by gradual tapering of the original drug or its periodic substitution by another medication (i.e., drug "vacations").

Tolerance is also a normal, physiologic adaptation. Exposure of a drug over time can lead to diminution of one or more of the drug's effects, requiring more of the drug to achieve the same therapeutic effects. Drug vacations can help prevent or mitigate the development of drug tolerance.

Addiction is a primary, chronic, neurobiologic disease. Genetic, psychosocial, and environmental factors influence its development and manifestations. Addiction is characterized by compulsive behaviors at a functional level and continued use of the drug despite adverse consequences. Tolerance with prolonged use and withdrawal effects with cessation suggest physical dependence, not addiction.

Pseudoaddiction is an iatrogenic syndrome of drug-seeking behavior due to inadequate pain management. It is characterized by demands for dose escalations by the patient. It can possibly lead to true addiction. With adequate treatment of pain, pseudo-addiction ceases, but addiction continues.

Aberrant drug-seeking behaviors include unsanctioned drug dosage escalations, losing prescriptions on a regular basis, prescription forgery, concurrent abuse of illicit substances, and medication diversion. These behaviors may be due to either addiction or pseudoaddiction (which may precede a full-blown addiction). Identifying questionable behaviors as "drug misuse" prevents premature use of a diagnostic label. The differential diagnosis also includes depression, anxiety, organic mental syndrome, borderline personality disorder, other psychiatric disorders, and criminal intent.

History - All relevant medical history and referral info should be reviewed, including medical reports, educational and employment history, and substance abuse history of patient and his/her family and other relations. Special attention should be paid to reports of trauma, hepatitis, HIV infection, GI ulceration, history of multiple drug allergies, and diagnoses for which there are no objective clinical findings (e.g., trigeminal neuralgia). Patients with addiction sometimes have a history of unsatisfactory interactions with physicians and numerous missed appointments.

Most people in recovery will discuss their addictions, but patients practicing abstinence-only may not; both groups are at risk of relapse in the course of treatment for pain conditions.

Physical exam and objective signs - Look for cutaneous stigmata and other skin findings, psychomotor, neurologic signs, and lab abnormalities of drug and alcohol abuse (e.g., increased γGT and mean cell volume). Also look for increased sympathetic activity due to pain exacerbation. Increased sympathetic activity during withdrawal from alcohol, opioids, or benzodiazepines, and sleep disturbance can exacerbate pain. In addition, any psychological, emotional, or social stress can exacerbate pain.

Treatment - There are, unfortunately, many factors that complicate the management of patients with pain and concomitant substance abuse, including:
• lack of objective ways of diagnosing and assessing pain or addiction;
• imprecise addiction terminology;
• difficulty separating true addiction from similar conditions;
• stigmatization leading to underdiagnosis and undertreatment of pain and substance abuse disorders;
• frequent concomitant psychological and medical disorders;
• complex effects of addiction on pain and vice versa;
• lack of a clear concensus for treatments;
• difficulty establishing trust with patients with addiction;
• litigation fears.

Myths and misconceptions regarding the pain in patients concomitantly abusing substances include the beliefs that:
• the pain is not real and the patient just wants to "get high";
• giving patients in pain narcotics will only increase addiction;
• in the setting of addiction, nothing will help with pain;
• when on methadone, narcotics are not needed for pain.

Pointers for treatment include:
- patients with addiction should receive the same standard pain management measures when appropriate (e.g., PCA or epidural analgesia) as for non-addicted patients;
- pain and addiction treatment must occur simultaneously; an agreement in writing about concrete and attainable goals helps clarify both the patient's and provider's responsibilities; these agreements must be strict contracts; regular urine toxicology screening should be pursued;
- cues for craving need to be minimized, e.g., minimize exposure to phlebotomy if possible (i.e., avoid unnecessary tests and have patients look away if tests have to be done);
- patients should be reminded of past problems from the abuse, as many abusers forget all their past dysfunctions and problems (Musto's theory);
- with increases in pain, encourage increasing contact with their sponsor or other healthy social supports; other trusted individuals, not the patient, should dispense the analgesic;
- select and prescribe drugs prudently (i.e., drugs with a lower abuse potential), using set schedules (around-the-clock; e.g., at 0800, 1400, and 2000, instead of TID); prescriptions should be written by only one prescriber;
- consider tolerance when prescribing drugs; regular reassessment of the adequacy of treatment are necessary; the focus should be on the patient's pain level, sedation, and functional status, not the number of milligrams given.

Urine toxicology screen (UTS)

Urine is a superior method in determining the presence or absence of certain drugs compared to blood, nails, or hair.
- Readily available, collected non-invasively.
- Easily handled by laboratory personnel.
- Increased window of detection (1–3 days for most drugs).
- Less invasive and less expensive than serum testing.

Fishbain et al. (2008) reviewed relevant literature and found the prevalence of addictive disorders in patients on long-term opioid treatment to be 3.27% and aberrant drug-related behavior/illicit drug use in the range of 11.5% to 20.4%.

Ives et al. (2006), in a prospective study, noted age, past cocaine abuse, drug or DUI conviction, and a past EtOH abuse as predictors of misuse. Race, income, education, depression score, disability score, pain score, and literacy were not associated with misuse. No relationship of pain score and misuse emerged.

When used with appropriate understanding, UTS can improve ability to manage controlled substance therapy, diagnose substance misuse/addiction, and serve as an advocate for patients. Patients who should be considered for testing include patients already taking controlled substances, patients being considered for prescription of controlled substances, patients resistant to full evaluation, patients requesting a specific drug(s), patients displaying aberrant behaviors, and patients in recovery. Written treatments are often necessary, and tests should be conducted when any aberrant drug-related behavior is noted or when a third party reports about aberrant drug related behaviors (family, friends, insurers, law enforcements, etc.). Random collection is preferred. Unobserved collection is usually acceptable, although if tampering is suspected, confirm that temperature is 90–100° F, creatinine >20mg/dL, and pH 4.5–8.0.

Confirmatory testing with *HPLC (high performance liquid chromatography), AxSYM, Rapid One Oxy*, and *Immunoassays* report each sample as positive or negative for particular drug/class and may be necessary.

Positive UTS results reflect recent drug use. UTS does not determine exposure time, dose, or frequency of use. Clinical urine testing, like any other medical tests, is performed to improve patient care and safety. Inappropriate interpretation may adversely affect care, as can premature discontinuance of opioids therapy secondary to no detection of opioids in urine. UTS and opioid testing should be used in conjunction with other clinical information and in close consultation with clinical toxicologist regarding results. "No Drug Detected" may mean that the patient does not or has not recently used drug; excretes drug/ metabolite faster than normal; UTS used is not sufficiently sensitive to detect the drug at concentration present; or that there is a clerical error.

Understanding how a drug metabolizes helps determine validity of a test. For example, codeine is metabolized to morphine. Hence, prescribed codeine may explain presence of both drugs (codeine & morphine) in urine. However, prescription of morphine does not explain presence of codeine. Codeine alone is possible in patients who lack hepatic enzyme CYP2D6. Also, cross-reaction with structurally similar prescription drugs for Parkinson's disease, over-the-counter diet agents and decongestants may occur. For instance, drugs such as selegiline, benzphetamine, clobenzorex, dimethyamphetamine, fenproporex, and mefenorex metabolize to amphetamine/metamphetamine. Proton pump inhibitors (pantoprazole) may affect immunoassays leading to false positive test for marijuana. Cannabinoids are not usually detected in the urine after only passive inhalation, but can be detected in the urine after cessation of MJ use for up to 80 days in a heavy user.

UTS results must be investigated carefully because some of the tests have been shown to have poor sensitivity and specificity, have a high incidence of false positive results, and be inadequate to meet the needs of pain physicians. Inter-patient variability in metabolism could show an absence of substance in the urine despite adherence and proper use. Changing laboratory threshold values (cutoff value) may affect what is reported as positive or negative.

Poppy seeds contain small amounts of morphine and codeine. Ingestion of food products containing poppy seeds can result in a positive urine test result.

Ref: Savage SR, et al. Definitions related to the medical use of opioids: evolution towards universal agreement. *J Pain Symptom Manage* 2003;26:655; **Fishbain DA, et al.** What Percentage of Chronic Nonmalignant Pain Patients Exposed to Chronic Opioid Analgesic Therapy Develop Abuse/Addiction and/or Aberrant Drug-Related Behaviors? A Structured Evidence-Based Review. *Pain Medicine.* 2008;9:444; **Ives TJ, et al.** Predictors of opioid misuse in patients with chronic pain: a prospective cohort study. *BMC Health Services Research* 2006;6:46.

Ch.22: CANCER PAIN

Pain relief is integral to the care of cancer patients at all stages of illness. Cancer pain can be due to direct effects (e.g., invasion of bone by tumor, nerve compression), complications of treatment (e.g., radiation fibrosis, chemotherapy-related neuropathy), or unrelated causes (migraines, arthritis). Pain may be somatic, visceral, or neuropathic in nature.

Several common cancer pain syndromes are worth highlighting: 1) Osseous pain due to bony metastases; 2) Thoracic pain due to local invasion of intercostal nerves; 3) Nerve root compression; 4) Peripheral nerve compression; 5) Herpes zoster; and 6) Phantom limb syndrome. Cancer pain management includes nonpharmacologic strategies, appropriate use of pharmacologic agents, including both analgesics agents and various adjuvants, and interventional approaches. The physician must always assess the patient carefully, as there may be multiple pains with multiple origins and mechanisms.

Non-opioid Analgesics: NSAIDs and acetaminophen are first-line and should be used around the clock prior to starting opioids. Acetaminophen should be used cautiously in chronic cancer patients because of the risk of hepatotoxicity (alcohol use and starvation predispose to toxicity at low doses).

Opioid Therapy: Opioids are invaluable because of their reliability, safety, multiple routes of administration, and ease of titration. Opioids can be used for somatic, visceral, and neuropathic pain (although neuropathic pain can be more difficult to treat with opioids alone).

Initial agents: The "weak" opioids (codeine, hydrocodone, oxycodone) can be combined with NSAIDs or acetaminophen and are effective for mild to moderate pain. Tramadol, a synthetic analog of codeine, may have a dual mechanism of action by binding to the mu-opioid receptor and inhibiting neuronal reuptake of serotonin and norepinephrine. Tramadol is useful for mild to moderate pain in patients who do not tolerate typical opioids but should be avoided in patients predisposed to seizures.

Use in renal failure: Avoid meperidine (Demerol; active metabolite, normeperidine, can cause CNS excitability), morphine (metabolite can lead to active narcosis), and codeine or tramadol (can accumulate and reduce seizure threshold). Methadone and fentanyl patch are considered best choices in those with renal failure (Dean, 2004).

Initiation of therapy: Typically start with a short-acting opioid every 2–3 hours as needed. Increase the dose by 25% to 50% until adequate analgesia is achieved. A long-acting opioid is then substituted. An additional short-acting opioid (equal to 10% to 20% of the total 24-hour opioid dose) should be available every 1–3 hours for breakthrough pain. If the breakthrough medication is needed more than 3 times a day, the amount of the long-acting opioid is increased.

Route of administration: Oral dosing may not be feasible in patients with oral mucositis, dysphagia, bowel obstruction, or severe nausea. Alternatives include: 1) rectal administration (morphine, oxymorphone, hydromorphone) but variations in drug bioavailability makes consistent analgesia difficult; 2) Transdermal (fentanyl only). Onset of analgesia is 12–14 hours from application; 3) Oral transmucosal fentanyl "lollipop" or concentrated solutions of morphine, oxycodone, or hydromorphone made by specialized pharmacists; and 4) Parenteral if other routes not feasible or rapid dose titration is required. Patient controlled analgesia provides analgesia that is the same or better than nurse-administered opioids with lower total opioid consumption and fewer side effects.

Management of opioid side effects: Approaches include: 1) dose reduction; 2) changing to a different opioid or route of administration; or 3) managing side effects symptomatically (nausea and vomiting, constipation, sedation, respiratory depression, myoclonus, pruritus).

Analgesic Adjuvants: Useful to provide an opioid-sparing effect and treating neuropathic pain.

Antidepressants: Tricyclic antidepressants modulate sodium channels and may also have alpha-2 agonist activity. They are helpful in neuropathic pain (e.g., burning, searing, aching, or dysesthetic pain in setting of known or probable nerve injury). Trazodone and SSRIs are not as effective for neuropathic pain but may be useful for patients with cancer pain with coexisting depression.

Anticonvulsants: May be very useful in the treatment of neuropathic pain. Agents include phenytoin, gabapentin, carbamazepine, valproic acid, clonazepam.

Sedatives and tranquilizers: Benzodiazepines and barbiturates have no significant analgesic effect, but may be valuable in reducing the anxiety associated with uncontrolled pain and cancer.

Local anesthetics: (e.g., topical lidocaine) used for treatment of mucocutaneous and neuropathic pain.

Bisphosphonates and calcitonin: Role of bisphosphonates for bone pain is unclear with mixed results based on clinical trials. Calcitonin provides no benefit for metastatic bone pain based on a Cochrane analysis (Martinez-Zapata, 2006).

Corticosteroids: Used as an analgesic when inflammation or vasogenic edema causes pain (neural compression, bony and soft tissue infiltration, visceral distension, etc.).

Capsaicin: May help control pain from oral mucositis, postmastectomy pain, and postherpetic neuralgia.

Clonidine: An alpha-2 receptor agonist, may be a useful analgesic adjuvant for opioids, especially for neuropathic pain.

Non-pharmacologic therapy of cancer pain: *Psychological approaches* include psychotherapy, and cognitive-behavioral therapy. They can help the patient cope with the illness and its symptoms. They are most useful for pain that is predictable, incidental pain.

Physical modalities: Useful for mild to moderate pain and often overlooked. Include cold, heat, exercise, and TENS (especially useful for phantom limb and post-thoracotomy pain syndromes).

Radiation therapy: Valuable in management of painful bone metastases.

Radiofrequency ablation: Applies thermal energy to individual tumor lesions which cannot be treated with surgery or radiation. Can provide relief for refractory bone metastases pain and possibly in soft tissue pain.

Interventional procedures: If pain is inadequately controlled with the above measures or side effects are intolerable, the patient may be a candidate for an inva-

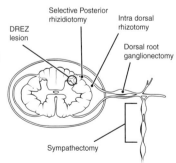

sive anesthetic or neurosurgical procedure. Epidural or intrathecal injection of opioids and local anesthetics can prove very useful. Nerve blocks using a local anesthetic, corticosteroid, or neurolytic agent can control intractable pain related to a nerve structure. Examples of nerve blocks for tumor infiltration include a celiac block (upper abdominal organs), hypogastric block (pelvic organs), stellate ganglion block (head and neck), and lumbar sympathetic block (leg). Examples of neurosurgical procedures include dorsal root entry zone (DREZ) lesioning, selective posterior rhizidiotomy, intra dorsal rhizotomy, dorsal root ganglionectomy and sympathectomy (see figure).

Ref: Bajwa ZH and Warfield CA. Pharmacologic Therapy of Cancer Pain. UptoDate. May 2006; **King LA and Billings JA.** Management of Chronic Cancer Pain. Primary Care Medicine, 4th ed. Goroll, AH, Mulley AG, eds. 2000; **Dean M.** Opioids in renal failure and dialysis patients. *J Pain Sympt Mgmt* 2004;28:497; **Martinez-Zapata MJ, et al.** Calcitonin for metastatic bone pain. *Cochrane Database Syst Rev* 2006;(3):CD003223.

Ch.23: ULTRASOUND GUIDED INJECTIONS

Ultrasound technology is a well-established radiology tool that allows physicians to perform image-guided soft tissue and joint injections without the use of ionizing radiation associated with x-ray or CT. Studies have noted enhanced patient comfort when ultrasound guidance is used for various injections (Marhofer, 2004; O'Sullivan, 2008; Shankar 2008). In addition, research of ultrasound guided injections has shown improved accuracy and efficiency in peripheral nerve blockade, soft tissue injections, and joint injections (Orenbaugh, 2007; Cimmino, 2008). Physicians are also utilizing ultrasound as an extension of a dynamic and functional musculoskeletal physical examination. While CT and MRI scans have superior static images, ultrasound can be performed while the patient demonstrates a painful movement, i.e., a painful shoulder arc range of motion, illuminating muscle patterns such as impingements. Studies have also examined performing epidural steroid injections under ultrasound guidance (Klocke, 2003; Kim, 2008).

Ultrasound images have been combined with electrodiagnostic examination findings. For example, in the diagnosis of carpal tunnel syndrome, dynamic nerve movements of the median nerve have been observed as it travels through the carpal tunnel. Beginning research is yielding normal values for median nerve and carpal tunnel measurements (Walker, 2004; Warner, 2004).

Research in areas of ultrasound-guided injections is ongoing. Number of physicians incorporating ultrasound-guided injections appears to be on the rise. Steep learning curve associated with interpreting ultrasound image is a potential barrier.

Ref: Shankar H. Ultrasound-guided steroid injection for obturator neuralgia. *Pain Pract.* 2008 Jul-Aug;8(4):320; **Orebaugh SL, et al.** Ultrasound guidance with nerve stimulation reduces the time necessary for resident peripheral nerve blockade. *Reg Anesth Pain Med* 2007;32:448; **Cimmino MA, et al.** Modern imaging techniques: a revolution for rheumatology practice. *Best Prac Res Clin Rheum* 2008;22:951; **Marhofer P, et al.** Ultrasound guidance for infraclavicular brachial plexus anaesthesia in children. *Anaesthesia* 2004;59:642; **O'Sullivan MJ.** Patient comfort in regional anesthesia. *Anesth Analg* 2008;106:349; **Kim SH et al.** Sonographic estimation of needle depth for cervical epidural blocks. *Anesth Analg.* 2008;106:1542; **Klocke R, et al.** Sonographically guided caudal epidural steroid injections. *J Ultrasound Med* 2003;22:1229; **Walker FO.** Imaging nerve and muscle with ultrasound. *Suppl Clin Neurophysiol.* 2004;57:243; **Werner RA, et al.** Influence of body mass index on median nerve function, carpal canal pressure, and cross-sectional area of the median nerve. *Muscle Nerve* 2004;30:481.

Ch.24: EMERGENCIES

Symptomatic bradycardia (HR <60/min or significantly diminished from baseline):
• Options include: atropine 0.5 mg IV q3–5 min up to max 3 mg total; dopamine 2–10 mcg/kg/min; epinephrine 2–10 mcg/min; transcutaneous pacing

Symptomatic unstable tachycardia (ventricular rate >150/min; for ventricular tachycardia, paroxysmal supraventricular tachycardia, and atrial flutter):
• Open airway; chest compressions as necessary
• Positive-pressure ventilation
• Synchronized cardioversion 100, 200, 300, 360 J, sequentially

Stable narrow complex tachycardia (narrow QRS [<0.12 sec] and ventricular rate >150/min; stable, no serious symptoms):
• Regular rhythm: vagal maneuvers, adenosine 6 mg rapid IV push over 1–3 secs
• Irregular rhythm: possible atrial fibrillation, atrial flutter, or multifocal atiral tachycardia; consult medicine/cardiology, control rate with diltiazem, beta-blockers (use with caution)

Wide complex (regular) tachycardia (wide QRS [>0.12 sec])
Ventricular tachycardia or uncertain rhythm:
• Amiodarone 150 mg IV over 10 mins, repeat prn to a max of 2.2 gm over 24 hrs; prepare for elective synchronized cardioversion
Supraventricular tachycardia with aberrant conduction:
• Adenosine 6 mg rapid IV push over 1–3 secs, followed by adenosine 12 mg IV push over 1–3 secs after 1–2 mins (may repeat once)

Wide complex (irregular) tachycardia (wide QRS [>0.12 sec])
Atrial fibrillation with aberrant conduction:
• Consult cardiology, control rate with diltiazem, beta-blockers (use with caution)
For atrial fibrillation + Wolf-Parkinson-White:
• Consult cardiology; avoid AV node blocking agents (adenosine, digoxin, diltiazem, verampamil); consider antiarrhythmics (e.g., amiodarone 150 mg IV over 10 mins)
• For ventricular rates ≤ 150/min, cardioversion generally not needed

Neurocardiogenic (vasovagal) syncope
• Restore to recumbent or Trendelenburg position; early recognition, restoration of recumbency, and reassurance are key

Anaphylaxis/lidocaine allergy
• 0.3–0.5 ml of epinephrine 1:1000 SQ, repeat q15 min prn; (pediatric dose 0.01 mL/kg up to 0.5 ml max)
• Prepare to initiate CPR if respiratory failure and shock follow; hospitalization for a 24 hr observation is advised

Acute myocardiac infarction
• Assess vitals, oxygen saturation; place IV; obtain EKG, CXR, electrolytes and coagulation profile; treatment is "MONA":
  • <u>M</u>orphine IV (if pain not relieved by nitroglycerin)
  • <u>O</u>xygen (4 L/min)
  • <u>N</u>itroglycerin SL
  • <u>A</u>spirin 160–325 mg p.o.

Cardiogenic Shock
- If problem is from heart pump failure and systolic BP <70, with signs/symptoms of shock: norepinephrine 0.5–30 mcg/min IV, then dopamine if needed
- If systolic BP 70–100 mm Hg with signs/symptoms of shock: dopamine 5–15 mcg/kg/min IV, then dobutamine if needed
- If systolic BP 70–100 mm Hg, and there are NO shock signs or symptoms: dobutamine 2–20 mcg/kg/min IV, then nitroglycerin if needed
- If systolic BP >100 mm Hg: nitroglycerin 10–20 mcg/min IV; consider nitroprusside 0.1–5.0 mcg/kg/min IV, then "3rd line actions" prn
- Defibrillate for ventricular fibrillation
- Consider lipid emulsion for local anesthetic-induced toxicity

Spinal cord injury (NASCIS protocols)
- Injury within 3 hrs: methylprednisolone 30 mg/kg over 45 mins, 15 mins rest, then 5.4 mg/kg/hr × 23 hrs
- Injury 3–8 hrs prior: methylprednisolone 30 mg/kg over 45 mins, 15 mins rest, then 5.4 mg/kg/hr × 47 hrs
- Note: although widely used, the above "mega-dose" steroid regimens are controversial; some do not consider the NASCIS protocols to be the standard of care (Hurlbert, 2000)

Ref: ACLS Provider Manual, American Heart Association, 2006; **Hurlbert RJ.** Methylprednisolone for acute spinal cord injury: an inappropriate standard of care. *J Neurosurg* 2000;93(S1):1.

INDEX